brush teeth regularly, fluoride treatments, change in taste sense, difficulty swallowing, hoarseness.

Neck : Stiffness, pain, masses.

Breasts, axillae : Discharge, bleeding, masses, changes with menses, breast self-examination.

Respiratory : Chest X-ray (date, result), wheezing, cough, hemoptysis, expectoration, dyspnea, night sweats, sneezing, rhinorrhea.

Cardiovascular : Dyspnea on exertion, orthopnea, paroxysmal nocturnal dyspnea, hypertension, claudication, varicose veins, thrombophlebitis, Raynaud's syncope, chest pain, palpitations, tachycardia, heart murmur, peripheral edema.

Gastrointestinal : Dietary habits, appetite, food intolerance, use of antacids, indigestion, nausea, vomiting, distention, abdominal pains, abdominal masses, jaundice, hematemesis, bowel habits, use of laxatives, constipation, melana, mucus in stools, acholic stools, tarry stools, diarrhea, hemorrhoids, incontinence, abdominal surgery.

Genitourinary : Male and female—Sexual habits, venereal disease, potency, dysuria, polyuria, oliguria, hematuria, pyuria, calculi, force of stream, retention, frequency, hesitancy, nocturia, incontinence, discharge. Male—prostatitis, hernia.

Gynecological : Menarche, duration, amount, interval, catamenia, menorrhagia, metrorrhagia, date last menstrual period, amenorrhea, type of contraception, infertility, dyspareunia, postcoital bleeding, vaginal discharge, pruritis, date and result of last Pap smear, vaginal or uterine surgery.

Obstetrical : Pregnancies, full-term deliveries, premature deliveries, abortions, living children, complications of pregnancies.

Musculoskeletal : Muscle weakness, pain, aches, cramps, atrophy, back or joint stiffness, pain, deformity, dislocation, fractures, radicular pain.

Neurologic : Headache, nervousness, sleep disturbance, vertigo, syncope, sensory or motor disturbance, paralysis/paresis, paresthesia/hyperesthesia/hypesthesia, memory loss, nightmares, twitching, convulsions, tremors, dysphagia, handwriting changes, loss of consciousness, disorientation.

Psychiatric : Disorientation, irritability, depression, mood swings, suicidal or homicidal attempts, delusions, hallucinations, feelings of persecution, ideas of reference, paranoia, anxiety, phobias, indecision, preoccupation, obsessive rumination.

Endocrine : Change in skin color or texture, hair distribution, sexual vigor, voice, goiter, polydipsia, polyphagia, polyuria, growth change, intolerance to temperature, sugar in blood or urine, excessive sweating.

Lymphatic and hematologic : Lymph node swellings, excessive bleeding, bruising, anemia, blood transfusions.

POCKET GUIDE TO

Health Assessment

Karen J. Berger, R.N., B.S.N., M.S.
Willa L. Fields, R.N., M.S.Ed.

RESTON PUBLISHING COMPANY, INC.
A Prentice-Hall Company
Reston, Virginia

Illustrations by Anita Yakeley

Library of Congress Cataloging in Publication Data

Berger, Karen J
    Pocket guide to health assessment.

    Includes bibliographical references and index.
    1.   Physical diagnosis—Outlines, syllabi, etc.
2.   Medical history taking—Outlines, syllabi, etc.
I.   Fields, Willa L., joint author, II.   Title.
[DNLM: 1. Diagnosis—Handbooks. WB141.3. B496p]
RC76.B47   616.07'5   79-14659
ISBN 0-8359-5582-6

10   9   8   7   6   5   4   3   2   1

Printed in the United States of America

Contents

Preface

The past few years have seen a proliferation of books on health assessment, creating a bewildering array of choices for the practitioner. Some of these books are designed for beginners and some for the more advanced; some are general and some more specialized. Almost all are textbook-sized and bulky, containing facts and information seemingly by the pound. In their bulk and form these volumes create a heavy load for mental ingestion, and the ingesting must take place before moving into the clinical setting, as such tomes do not avail themselves readily to quick-resource use.

By contrast, this reference contains a *comprehensive* item *inventory* on *health assessment*, yet its *concise outline form* allows for a convenient 5" x 8" size. It is intended as a *clinical support* for fast cueing of the primed memory, while the student or, indeed, the experienced practitioner applies skills in the clinical setting. Its role should be that of a *hip pocket checklist*, one aimed at *preventing* the *memory slips* which may complicate the assessment process.

In that regard, the book contains a listing of all the observations in the conventional physical examination. Each observation written in medical terminology is followed by a description of the normal finding and parameters helpful for differentiating the normal state. We have provided diagrams and charts to help in making clinical judgments and guidelines to record physical signs. At the end of each chapter is a section describing the variations in physical findings commonly associated with the transformations of the life cycle. This is followed by a listing of abnormal adult and pediatric conditions. The special observations of the young and old, therefore, are not ignored.

In addition, an outline of the screening health history is included. Chapter 1 outlines the conventional components item by item. In the chapters that follow, questions in the review of systems are listed with each section of the clinical examination. An interesting and important feature is that key phrases, stated in lay language, are suggested for the composition of history questions, and the correlated medical terms follow in parentheses. This approach should help the beginning student learn the translation to medical terminology, while assisting the postgraduate student and the clinician in avoiding the awkward tendency to speak "medicalese." Again, the history inventory reflects attention to the life-cycle variations in the special questions on childhood and retirement.

We wish to stress that this book is intended as a memory cueing tool only, not as a primary textbook. We hope it will prove helpful for beginning students in physical assessment who are not yet fully comfortable with their new skills. Students using this pocket reference, however, must have had thorough didactic training in the methods and content of the health history and the physical examination, for it contains few explanations, and no theories, principles, or procedures. For that purpose, a companion textbook is being prepared, which will expand into these areas and guide learning in health assessment, as this book guides practice.

We must emphasize that in no way is the use of this book limited to students. Indeed, it should serve as a well-rounded clinical tool for the clinician who does not wish to rely totally on the fallible human memory and who requires periodic help recalling the myriad details in health assessments.

Lawrence Weed, originator of the Problem Oriented Medical Record System, was one of the first to recognize the value and necessity of memory cueing devices in the medical field. The beginning primary care student should find this book a helpful aid for that most painful student malady, the "mental dumping" syndrome. And the practitioner who just requires a checklist should find this a helpful clinical assessment tool as well.

Karen J. Berger
Willa L. Fields

Acknowledgments

We wish to acknowledge the following persons for their assistance in editing this work, and, moreover, for the enthusiasm they expressed, and the encouragement they gave:

John A. Berger, M.D.
Karen M. Campbell, R.N.
Steven R. Drosman, M.D.
George W. Le Fevre, M.D.
Edward L. Fields, M.D.
Philip R. Franklin, M.D.
Frederick Frye, M.D.
Edward W. Gallagher, M.D.
Warren O. Kessler, M.D.
John R. Morse, M.D.
Jere J. Nelson, M.D.
Ralph R. Ocampo, M.D.
Constance Salerno, R.N.
Robert Scheeler, B.S.
Julio R. Veinbergs, M.D.
John B. Welsh, M.D.

1
Health History

The following information, elicited prior to the physical examination, will give the examiner a picture of the current health status of the client, his health practices, his present and past health problems, and information about the client as a person coping with his own world. The outline below sets out a systematic procedure for doing the conventional screening health history, and, as such, it is a tool to assist in avoiding omissions. Also, suggestions are made for phrasing questions in the interest of improving practitioner-client communication.

I. IDENTIFYING INFORMATION (ID)

A Name
B Address
C Telephone number
D Age
E Sex
F Race

G Nationality
H Marital status
I Occupation
J Social Security number
K Informant
L Reliability of historian

II. CHIEF COMPLAINT (CC)

A. ***Specific reason for seeking health care***: What problem has lead you to seek help? What brings you here today?
(*Note*: Record as a quotation.)

B. ***Duration of the problem***: How long have you had this problem?

III. HISTORY OF PRESENT ILLNESS (HPI): Tell me all you can about your problem (if any).
(*Note*: If there is no immediate problem make note and proceed to IV, Past Medical History.)

A. Details of onset

1. *Date*: When did you begin having trouble?
2. *Situation*: What were you doing at the time?
3. *Mode of onset*: Did it come on fast or slow?
4. *Precipitating events*: What seemed to bring on the problem?

B. Character of problem

1. *Location of symptoms*: Where do you feel the _____ (pain, burning, etc.)
2. *Quality of symptoms*: Describe the feeling.
3. *Severity of symptoms*: How bad is it?
4. *Manner of relief*: What do you do for relief?
5. *Duration of episode*: How long does the _____ (symptom) usually last?
6. *Association with other symptoms*: Do you notice any other symptoms associated with your problem?
7. *Relation to habits and activities*: Do your symptoms have any relation to anything you usually do?

C. Progress of problem

1. *Sequence of symptoms development*: In what order did your symptoms come on?
2. *Persistence of symptoms*: How long has the problem been troubling you?
3. *Recurrence*: Does the problem come back?
4. *Effect of treatments*: What effect does the treatment have?
5. *Changes in symptoms/behavior*: How have your symptoms changed?
6. *Effect of change in situation (if any)*: How did the change in situation effect the _____ (symptoms)?

D. Current status of problem

1. *Current symptoms*: Which symptoms are bothering you now?
2. *Location*: Where do you feel them?
3. *Severity*: How bad?

E. Client's interpretation of cause and effects of problem: What do you think is causing the problem? What effects has the problem had?

F. Reason the problem is of concern to the client: What about your problem troubles you most?

G. Reason for seeking help at present: What brings you to seek help now?

IV. PAST MEDICAL HISTORY (PMH): What illnesses have you had in the past?

A. Adult PMH:
(*Note*: Record all previous diagnoses with dates, severity, complications, how diagnosis established, place and length of hospitalization and/or convalescence, name of physician of record.

1. *Medical illnesses*?
2. *Operations* (surgical procedures)? Complications?
3. *Transfusions*?
4. *Psychiatric illnesses*?
5. *Hospitalization*?
6. *Childhood diseases*: Chicken pox? Diphtheria? Measles? Tetanus? Mumps? Polio? Rheumatic fever? Rubella? Scarlet fever? Strept throat? Whooping cough? Mononucleosis? Any sequalae?
7. *Immunizations*: DPT? TOPV? MMR? Small Pox? Typhoid? Boosters? Reactions? TB skin tests?
8. *Injuries*? Nature of accident? How happened? Wear seat belts? Use firearms? Disabilities?
9. *Allergies*? Hay fever? Asthma? Reaction to food, drugs, contact agents, animals? Detailed description of reaction? Diagnosed by whom?

A. *Adult SH cont.*

10. *Current medications* (prescribed and over-the-counter)?
    Name? Dose? Schedule? Duration? Reason? Vitamins?

B. *Pediatric PMH*:
   (*Note*: Includes the above and the special areas below.)

1. *Prenatal*
    a.   Number pregnancies of mother?
    b.   Number living children?
    c.   Number miscarriages and stillborns?
    d.   Prenatal care during pregnancy? When begun? Where?
    e.   Infections during pregnancy? What month?
    f.   Other maternal illnesses during pregnancy? When? How treated?
    g.   X-rays during pregnancy? When? What type? Reason?
    h.   Injuries? When? How treated?
    i.   Medications during pregnancy? What kind? When? Reason?
    j.   Usual diet? Special diet? Reason?
    k.   Bleeding during pregnancy? Transfusions necessary?
    l.   Blood type? Rh negative?
    m.   Did pregnancy last 9 months (full-term)? If not, reason?

2. *Delivery*
    a.   How long was labor? What type delivery (vaginal, Caesarean)?
    b.   Anesthesia or other medications during delivery? Any problems? Need forceps?
    c.   Baby born where?
    d.   Birth weight?
    e.   Condition at birth? Blue? Cry? Need oxygen?

3. *Neonatal*
    a.   Baby have problems during hospital stay? Jaundice? Need oxygen? Incubator? Blood transfusion? Seizures?
    b.   Length of baby's hospital stay? Did baby and mother go home together?
    c.   Feeding problems during hospitalization?
    d.   How much weight did baby lose?
    e.   Rashes while in hospital?
    f.   Breast fed? Bottle fed?

4. *Developmental*
   a. Good eater? Accept new foods easily? Colic? Ease of going to sleep? Cried a lot? Wakeful? Vitamins? Iron? Fluoride? Tetracycline?
   b. Age smiled?
   c. Age head stable?
   d. Age sat alone?
   e. Age turned over?
   f. Age crept?
   g. Age walked alone?
   h. Age weaned?
   i. First tooth?
   j. First word?
   k. Toilet trained (bowel and bladder control)? Day? Night?
   l. Bed wetting (enuresis)?
   m. Sleep walking (somnambulism)?
   n. Development similar to or different from other children in family?
   o. Parent's overall evaluation of child's health?

V. FAMILY HISTORY (FH)

A. *Age and health status*, or age of death and cause, of parents, siblings, and children. Include grandparents in the case of pediatric clients or acknowledged familial disease.
   (*Note*: record as family tree chart. See fig. 1-1 on p. 6.)

B. *Family health status*: Allergy? Anemia? Arthritis? Asthma? Bleeding disorder? Cancer? Congenital malformation? Diabetes? Epilepsy? Genetic disorder? Glaucoma? Gout? Heart disease? Hypertension? Kidney disease? Mental illness? Obesity? Rheumatic fever? Stroke? TB? Ulcer? Arteriosclerosis? Depression?

VI. PERSONAL AND SOCIAL HISTORY (P/SH)

A. *Adult SH*

   1. *Vocational*
      a. Type of work? Currently employed? Where? Position? Duties? Happy with work? Recent change?

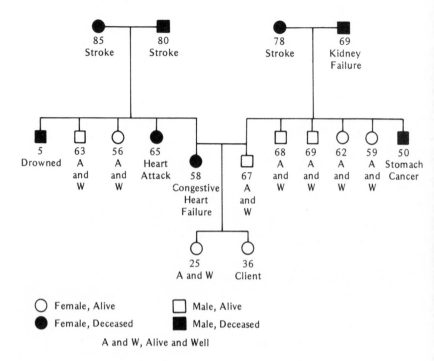

Figure 1-1   Recording the family history

b.   Exposure to hazardous agents? Asbestos? X-rays? Solvents?
     Radioactive substances?
c.   Job performance affected by illness?
d.   Years of schooling? High school diploma? College degree?
     Performance in school?
e.   Military history? Overseas assignment? Duties?
f.   Leisure activities? Exercise? Hobbies? Volunteer work?
g.   Financial status? Own or rent home? Unusual expenses
     (e.g., college tuition payments)? Savings? Health insurance?
     Disability insurance? Sick leave from work? Possible financial
     problems from illness?
h.   Retired? Attitude toward retirement? How coping?

A. Adult SH cont.

2. *Family*
   a. Locale of parents, siblings, children?
   b. Number of children?
   c. Who lives in home?
   d. Dependent parents, siblings, children?
   e. Describe home life. Satisfactory? If not, reason? Home life affected by illness? How?
   f. Type of housing? Number of rooms?

3. *Marital*
   a. Marital status? Length of time married? Happily married?
   b. Reason for separation or divorce?
   c. Age of spouse? State of health?
   d. Describe relationship. Satisfactory? If not, reason? Relationship affected by illness? How?

4. *Sexual*
   a. Sex education? Obtained where?
   b. Sexual orientation (heterosexual, homosexual, bisexual)?
   c. Present sex life satisfactory? If not, reason? Sexual performance or satisfaction affected by illness? How?
   d. Reach a climax (orgasm)?
   e. Use birth control? Type?

5. *Social*
   a. Describe social life. Social relationships satisfying? If not, reason? Social relationships affected by illness? How?
   b. Membership in social groups, clubs, or other organizations?
   c. Practice a religion? Religious preference?

6. *Habits*
   a. Tobacco:
      1. Smoke? What? Age started?
      2. Ever quit? For how long?
      3. How much?
         (*Note*: Record as pack-years for cigarettes.)

A. Adult SH cont.

  b. Alcohol

    1. Drink alcoholic beverages (beer, wine, whiskey, gin, others)?

    2. How much in average day, week, month?

    3. What time of day?

    4. Ever pass out from drinking (blackout)?

    5. Ever had DT's (delerium tremens)?

    6. Ever told by doctor to stop drinking? Reason?

    7. Arrested for drunk driving?

    8. Drinking ever caused problems at home or work?

  c. Other drugs of abuse

    1. Non-narcotic pain pills? Aspirin? Darvon? Empirin?

    2. Sleeping pills (sedatives and hypnotics)? Barbiturates? Quaalude? Doriden? Dalmane? Chloral hydrate?

    3. Diet or mood-elevating pills (antidepressants)? Amphetamines? Ritilin? Elavil?

    4. Nerve pills (tranquilizers)? Valium? Librium? Miltown?

    5. Hallucinogenic drugs? LSD?

    6. Marijuana?

    7. Cocaine?

    8. Narcotics? Heroin? Morphine? Dilaudid? Codeine?

    9. Others?

    10. Manner of use?

      a. Obtained through doctor's prescription? If not, how?

      b. Reason for taking?

      c. Quantity consumed per day?

      d. Route of administration?

  d. Nonalcoholic beverages

    1. Coffee or tea? Brand? Quantity per day?

    2. Cola? Quantity per day?

 7. *Geographic Exposure*: Areas of birth, residence, and travel?

 8. *Psychological/Psychiatric*

  a. Coping mechanisms

    1. Usual sources of worry, anxiety, doubts?

    2. Usual ways of achieving relief or feeling of well-being?

    3. Usual ways of handling crisis? Self? Family?

    b. Self image/body image: Describe feelings about self.

    c. Ever had psychological counseling or been under psychiatric care?

    d. For what? When? How long? Therapist?

    e. Any one in family ever had psychological counseling or been treated by a psychiatrist?

    f. Who? What age? When? Type of care?

9. *Activities of daily living*: Detailed activities throughout a typical day?

10. *Diet*: Detailed diet throughout a typical day?

B. Pediatric SH:
(Note: Following information asked of parents when client is young child, for adolescent refer also to adult social history.)

1. *Information on parents*
    a. Occupation? Both work? Hobbies? Educational level?
    b. Marital status?
    c. Financial status? Means of support adequate?
    d. Habits?

2. *Living situation*
    a. Both parents in the home?
    b. Extended family? Anyone else live in home?
    c. Type housing? Number of rooms? Child have own room?
    d. Adequate play facilities?
    e. Child care arrangements?

3. *Family relationships*
    a. Number of children in household?
    b. Position of child in family (birth order)?
    c. Relationship between children?
    d. Competition between children (sibling rivalry)? How handled?
    e. Describe parent-child relationship. Relationship satisfactory? (A specific inquiry should be made about parent of opposite sex in oedipal-age children.) If not, reason?
    f. Describe child's relationship with other family members. Relationship satisfactory? If not, reason?

B. *Pediatrics SH cont.*

      g.   Family organized satisfactorily for carrying out responsibilities of living (role organization)?

      h.   Who disciplines the child? Methods of discipline?

      i.   Anyone sick in family? Who?

      j.   Anyone in family in institution of any kind?

  4. *School and activities*

      a.   Grade?

      b.   Get along at school (social adaptation)?

      c.   Performance in school (educational achievement)?

      d.   Extracurricular and leisure activities? Hobbies?

      e.   Sex education? What? By whom?

  5. *Peer relationships*

      a.   Get along?

      b.   Adequate in number?

  6. *Activities of daily living:* Detailed activities during a typical day?

  7. *Diet*: Detailed diet throughout a typical day?

VII. REVIEW OF SYSTEMS (ROS):

(*Note*: Questions in lay terminology included with each representative section of the physical examination.)

A. *General*: Overall state of health, ability to carry out activities of daily living, weight changes, fatigue, exercise tolerance, fever, night sweats, repeated infections?

B. *Integument*: Change in skin pigmentation, texture or moisture, eruptions, rashes, pruritis, pain, unusual hair growth or loss, deformities or disorders of nails?

C. *Head, face, scalp*: Headache, trauma, sinus pain, scalp itching, scalp infestations?

D. *Eyes:* Visual problems, diplopia, scotomata, use of glasses, use of contact lenses, date of examination, eye pain, eye itching, lid edema, excessive tearing, tests for glaucoma, photophobia?

E. *Ears:* Mastoiditis, pain, discharge, tinnitus, dizziness, vertigo, hearing problem, sensitive to certain types of noise?

F. *Nose, mouth, and throat:* Smell, sinusitis, epistaxis, nasal obstruction, trauma, pain, discharge, head colds, fit of dentures, last visit to dentist, dental problems, pain, lesions, soreness of tongue, bleeding or swelling of gums, brush teeth regularly, fluoride treatments, change in taste sense, difficulty swallowing, hoarseness?

G. *Neck:* Stiffness, pain, masses, motion limited?

H. *Breasts and axillae:* Discharge, bleeding, masses, changes with menses, breast self-examination?

I. *Respiratory:* Chest X-ray (date, result), wheezing, cough, hemoptysis, expectoration, dyspnea, sneezing, rhinorrhea, night sweats?

J. *Cardiovascular:* Dyspnea on exertion, orthopnea, paroxysmal nocturnal dyspnea, hypertension, claudication, varicose veins, thrombophlebitis, Raynaud's, syncope, chest pain, palpitations, tachycardia, heart murmur, peripheral edema?

K. *Gastrointestinal:* Dietary habits, appetite, food intolerance, use of antacids, indigestion, nausea, vomiting, distention, abdominal pain, abdominal masses, jaundice, hematemesis, bowel habits, use of laxatives, constipation, melena, mucus in stools, acholic stools, tarry stools, diarrhea, hemorrhoids, incontinence? Abdominal surgery?

L. *Genitourinary:* Male and female—Sexual habits, venereal disease, potency, dysuria, polyuria, oliguria, hematuria, pyuria, calculi, force of stream, retention, frequency, hesitancy, nocturia, incontinence, discharge? Male—prostatitis, hernia?

M. *Gynecological:* Menarche (menses duration, amount, interval), catamenia, menorrhagia, metrorrhagia, date of last menstrual period, amenorrhea, type of contraception (if any), infertility, dyspareunia, postcoital bleeding, vaginal discharge, pruritis, date and result of last Pap smear, vaginal or uterine surgery?

N. *Obstetrical:* Pregnancies, full-term deliveries, premature deliveries, abortions, living children, complications of pregnancies?

O. *Musculoskeletal*: Muscle weakness, pain, aches, cramps, or atrophy, back or joint stiffness, pain, deformity, dislocation, fractures; radicular pain?

P. *Neurologic*: Headache, nervousness, sleep disturbance, vertigo, syncope, sensory or motor disturbance, paralysis/paresis, paresthesia, hypersthesia, hypesthesia, memory loss, nightmares, twitching, convulsions, tremors, dysphagia, handwriting changes, loss of consciousness, disorientation?

Q. *Psychiatric*: Disorientation, irritability, depression, mood swings, suicidal or homicidal attempts, delusions, hallucinations, feelings of persecution, ideas of reference, paranoia, anxiety, phobias, indecision, preoccupation, obsessive rumination, compulsion?

R. *Endocrine*: Change in skin color or texture, hair distribution, sexual vigor, voice, goiter, polydipsia, polyphagia, polyuria, growth change, intolerance to temperature, sugar in blood or urine, excessive sweating?

S. *Lymphatic and hematologic*: Lymph node swellings, excessive bleeding or bruising, anemia, blood transfusions?

2
General Survey

I. HISTORY QUESTIONS:
(*Note*: This section incorporates aspects of endocrine and hematologic histories.)

A   Overall health?

B   Gained or lost weight? Reason?

C   Appetite change? Always hungry (polyphagia)? Lost interest in eating (anorexia)?

D   Recent change in play or activity pattern?

E   Exhausted or fatigued most of the time?

F   Difficulty falling or staying asleep (insomnia)?

G   Fevers or periodic sweating, especially at night? Excessive sweating?

H   Change in size of hands or feet (acromegaly)?

I   Intolerance to weather changes (temperature intolerance)?

J   Thirsty a lot (polydipsia)?

K   Sugar in blood or urine (hyperglycemia, glycosuria)?

L   Repeated infections?

M   Ever had anemia?

N   Ever had blood transfusions?

II. CLINICAL EXAMINATION

A. *Preparation*

1. *Position*: Client comfortable. Infant or young child prone on adult's lap for rectal temperature and supine on measuring board for height.

2. *Equipment*: Watch with second hand, thermometer, sphygmo-menometer, stethoscope, scale with measuring arm, and measuring tape.

B. Inspection

1. *Mental status*? (NL* alert, orientated, behavior appropriate for age and situation)
2. *Presenting appearance*? (NL adequate hygiene, dress appropriate to situation, no obvious acute physical distress).
3. *Apparent sex*? (NL gender characteristics, hair distribution, body build, appropriate to sex)
4. *Apparent race*?
5. *Apparent age*? (NL apparent age correlates closely with stated age.)
6. *Nutrition*? (NL weight appropriate to height, age, and dietary intake. No obesity or emaciation. See height and weight tables for adults, Appendix I, and physical growth charts, Appendix II.)
7. *Body development*? (NL appropriate to age and consistent with genetic heritage, no gigantism or dwarfism, no acromegaly.)
8. *Body proportions*? (NL measurement from top of head to symphysis pubis equals measurement from symphysis pubis to floor, arm span equals height within 2 inches (5 centimeters). Proportions consistent with genetic heritage, endomorphic, ectomorphic, or mesomorphic.)
9. *Station/posture*? (NL flexible posture appropriate to activity and situation. Not fixed.)
10. *Body movement*? (NL appropriate to activity and situation. No involuntary movement.)
11. *Gait*? (NL fluid, balanced, coordinated walking movements. No unusually short steps, wide-based walk, restricted swinging of arms, staggering, trunkal lurching, dragging of feet, or watching feet while walking.)
12. *Cerebral dominance (handedness, sidedness)*? (NL consistent dominance pattern.)
13. *Energy level*? (NL able to persist in activity appropriate to situation without obvious fatigue, faltering, or difficulty in self-restraint.)

*NL: Normal

14. *Speech*? (NL fluent, well-articulated speech in language of facility. Speech patterns appropriate to age. No hoarseness, nasality, dysarthria, weakness.)
15. *Breath odors*? (NL no odor of ammonia, acetone, methyl mercaptan, ethanol, or other offensive smell.)

C. *Palpation*: Pulse? (NL 60-100 beats per minute. Strong and regular.)

D. *Percussion*: Not part of conventional general survey.

E. *Auscultation:* Blood pressure? (NL see blood pressure charts, Appendix III for adults; Appendix IV for various ages.)

F. *Measurements*
1. *Height*? (NL see height and weight tables for adults, Appendix I, physical growth charts, Appendix II.)
2. *Weight*? (NL see height and weight tables for adults, Appendix I, physical growth charts, Appendix II.)
3. *Temperature*? (NL oral 98.6°F. (37°C), and varies from 96.4° (35.7°C) in early morning, to 99.1° (37.3°C) in late afternoon. Rectal average 0.7° to 0.9°F higher than oral.)
4. *Pulse*? (NL 60-100 beats per minute in adults.)
   For children, see normal pulse rates for various ages, Appendix V.
5. *Blood pressure*? (NL see blood pressure charts, Appendix III, IV.)
6. *Respirations*? (NL see respiratory rate chart, Appendix II.)

III. LIFE-CYCLE VARIATIONS IN PHYSICAL FINDINGS

A. *Developmental*: Gait, balance, and stance vary with age in early childhood. Children aged 12-18 months show wide-stanced gait, little balance, poor ankle stability, though most progress to running by 18 months. Walking alone apparent by 21 months for an evaluation of normal. Speech development begins by age 3-4 months with babbling, cooing, and laughing; imitative vocalization by 9 months, and word formation appears by 1 year. All sounds should be articulated correctly by age 7. Newborn posture is one of partial flexion, changing by age 4 months to a symmetrical position. Infant head is large in relato body size, and reaches almost adult size by age 5 years. From age 1 on, head decreases in proportionate size. Secondary sex characteristics should be obvious by age 13 in girls and age 14 in boys. Height and weight are a function of age; see physical growth charts, Appendix II. Body fat decreases from age 1-6 in both sexes, followed by a period of subcutaneous fat accumulation, then proceeding to a bony growth spurt in early adolescence for almost all girls and two-thirds of the boys. For vital sign changes in normal childhood see normal blood pressure for various ages, Appendix IV, normal pulse rates for various ages, Appendix V, and normal respiratory rates for various ages, Appendix VI.

B.   *Degenerative*: Gait changes are evident in many elderly from a variety of abnormal neuromuscular and orthopedic conditions, though no specific change (except perhaps a slowing of gait) is associated solely with the aging process in the absence of frank disease. Body proportions change with aging, including a loss in height. By age 80 a loss of 3 inches (7.5 centimeters) from the adult peak is not uncommon, arm span increasing relative to overall height, as long bones retain their length. Neck and trunkal shortening occur in association with spinal shrinkage. Body fat often accumulates in the 5th and 6th decades, and may show redistribution with a loss over face, arms, legs, and back, and an increase over abdomen and hips. Speech may be altered slightly by loss of dentition or ill-fitting dentures, and response latency may increase in the elderly as speech discrimination ability declines. For blood pressure variations consistent with normal aging see adult blood pressure chart, Appendix III.

IV. ABNORMAL CONDITIONS

A.   *Pediatric*: Anemia, congenital heart defects, diabetes mellitus, hydrocephalus, leukemia, muscular dystrophy, nephritis, nephrosis, rheumatic heart disease, tuberculosis.

B.   *Adult*: Acromegaly, cirrhosis, depression, diabetes mellitus, emphysema, hypothyroidism, multiple sclerosis, tuberculosis.

3
Integument

I. HISTORY QUESTIONS

A Skin itchy (pruritus)? Where? Associated with what? Date of onset?
B Skin pain? Where? Associated with what? Date of onset?
C Rashes? Where? Associated with what? Date of onset?
D Recently bitten by mosquitoes? Fleas? Lice? Stinging insects? Anyone else in your household bitten?
E Exposed to anyone with scabies, impetigo, or other contagious skin condition?
F Recent hair loss (alopecia)? Recent unusual hair growth (hirsutism)? Change in consistency or feel of hair (texture)? Change in color of hair? Scalp itchy?
G Recent change in feel of skin? Oily (seborrhea)? Dry (xerosis)? Rough (scaling, crusting)?
H Recent change in mole color, size or sensitivity?
I Recent change in skin color? Loss of color (vitiligo)? Increased color (hyperpigmentation)?
J Recent change in nails? Shape? Color? Brittleness?
K Frequent bruising of skin?
L Family history of similar condition?

II. CLINICAL EXAMINATION

A. *Preparation*

1. *Position*: Client loosely draped and in a comfortable position.
2. *Equipment*: Adequate lighting, transparent ruler.

B. *Inspection*

    1. Skin

        a. Color? (NL appropriate to genetic heritage, no vitiligo, hyper-pigmentation, cyanosis, pallor, jaundice, carotinemia, erythema, mottling, or ashen appearance.)

        b. Consistency and texture? (NL moist, smooth, pores barely visible, not oily or dry, not scaly, crusty, or pig-skinned.)

        c. Hygiene? Body odor?

        d. Venous dilatation? Varicosities? (NL none.) Location?

        e. Edema? (NL none.) Pitting? Brawny? Location?

        f. Lesions? Primary? Secondary? Vascular? (See lesion charts and illustrations, tables 3-1, 3-2, 3-3, Fig. 3-1, 3-2.) (NL none.) Distribution? Location? Size? Contour? Consistency? Color?

        g. Masses? (NL none.)

        h. Bites? (NL none.) Insect? Animal? Human? Location? Appearance?

TABLE 3-1: Primary Skin Lesions

Term	Definition	Size	Example
macule	flat, nonpalpable colored spot	up to 5 mm	freckle
papule	solid elevated circumscribed lesion	up to 5 mm	acne
nodule	solid, elevated, circumscribed lesion	0.5-1.2 cm	eruthema nodosum
vesicle	fluid-filled, elevated, circumscribed lesion	up to 5 mm	herpes simplex
cyst	encapsulated, fluid-filled mass		epidermoid cyst
bulla	fluid-filled, elevated, circumscribed lesion	> 5 mm	severe poison ivy, pemphigus, 2nd-degree burn
pustule	pus-filled, elevated, circumscribed lesion	up to 5 mm	acne vulgaris
wheal	circumscribed, red white transient elevation	0.5 to 10 cm diameter	hives, urticaria, mosquito bite
tumor	solid, elevated mass	> 1 cm	cavernous hemangioma

TABLE 3-2:   Secondary Skin Lesions

Term	Definition	Example
scales	dried, thin, epithelial flakes of skin	psoriasis
crust	dried exudate	eczema, impetigo
fissures	crack in the skin usually extending through epidermis	chronic contact dermatitis, chapping
excoriation	self-produced traumatized area, scratch marks	eczema
ulcer	circumscribed area of destroyed epidermis, may extend into corium and subcutaneous tissue	stasis ulcer of varicose veins, chancre, malignant growth
scar	tibrotic area of dermus, caused by destruction of dermus and/or subcutaneous layers	healed surgical incision

TABLE 3-3:   Vascular Lesions

Term	Definition	Example
petechiae	tiny red or red brown capillary hemorrhages	idiopathic thrombocytopenic purpura
ecchymoses	hemorrhages under the skin	idiopathic thrombocytopenic purpura
telangiectasis	localized dilitation of individual superficial blood vessels	spider nevi associated with hepatocellular disease

2. *Hair*
   a. Color? Recent change?
   b. Texture? Recent change? (NL not brittle or dull.)
   c. Distribution? (NL appropriate to age and sex: See specific descriptions under each body region. No spotty alopecia or hirsutism.)
   d. Hygiene?

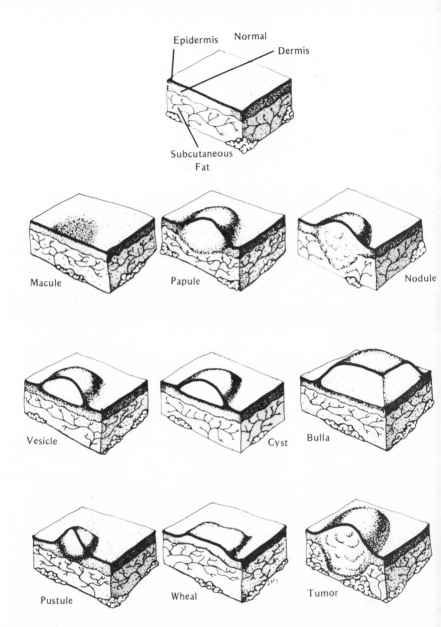

Figure 3-1 Primary skin lesions.

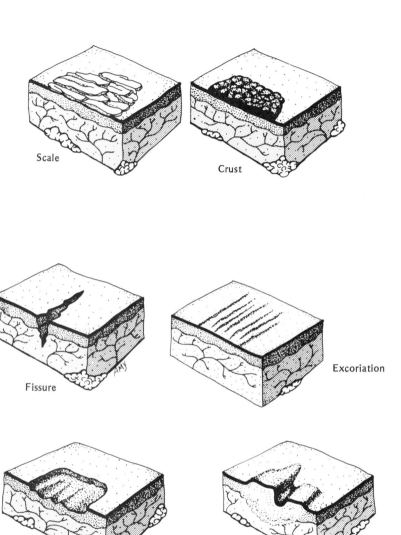

Scale

Crust

Fissure

Excoriation

Ulcer

Scar

Figure 3-2   Secondary skin lesions.

     3. Nails
-   *a.* Color? (NL translucent nail plate. No staining or discolorations.)
-   *b.* Consistency? (NL smooth, flexible. Not brittle or dry.)
-   *c.* Contour? (NL smooth, convex. No splitting, no Beau's lines, hypertrophy or subungual separation, clubbing or spooning.)
-   *d.* Hygiene?

C. *Palpation*

     1. Skin
-   *a.* Texture? (NL smoooth and firm. Not rough, oily.)
-   *b.* Moisture? (NL dry, but varies with environmental temperature and activity.)
-   *c.* Temperature? (NL evenly warm with little variance over body. Bilateral coolness on hands and feet normal.)
-   *d.* Elasticity? (NL elastic, on pinching recoils immediately to taut state.)
-   *e.* Pitting edema? (NL none.) Degree? Evaluation scale for recording pitting edema: 1+ edema barely detectable, 2+ indentation less than 5 mm, 3+ indentation less than 10 mm (1 cm), 4+ indentation greater than 10 mm (1 cm).
-   *f.* Masses? (NL none.) Location? Size? Contour? Consistency? Tenderness? Induration? Mobility? Boundaries?

     2. Nails: (NL flexible, no tenderness to compression.)

D. *Percussion and auscultation:* Not part of conventional integument examination.

III. LIFE CYCLE VARIATIONS IN PHYSICAL FINDINGS

A. *Developmental*

     1. Newborn: Epidermis thin, may show erythematous flush for first 24 hours of life, turning pale pink. Vasomotor changes in subcutaneous tissue may produce mottled appearance. Melanotic pigmentation not intense in black newborns. Physiological jaundice appears by day 2 or 3 of life and fades by 1 week, but may persist to 1 month. Fine downy hair, lanugo, covers entire body, and a cheesy white substance, vernix caseosa, is seen to varying degrees. Milia, tiny white raised areas, often appear over nose, cheeks, and forehead and represent retention of sebum in the opening of sebacious glands. Skin warm, moist, and elastic. Hair downy at first and gradually replaced by silky, fine hair which increases in thickness and density throughout childhood. Nails are very thin, peel easily, and gradually increase in hardness.

2. *Adolescence*: Scalp hair thick and dense. In male, occurrence of sparse downy pubic hair in a diamond shaped pattern occurs at age 10-14 years, becomes more heavily pigmented, dense, and curly over next 2-3 years. Axillary and facial hair appears at age 12-16 as sparse down and becomes more heavily pigmented and dense over the following year. In female pubic hair appears in the typical triangular pattern at age 8-13, axillary hair at age 9-14.

B. *Degenerative*

1. *Skin*: Loss of subcutaneous adipose and elasticity leads to decreased skin turgor and wrinkling. Some yellowish discoloration may be apparent in Caucasians. Areas of hyperpigmentation and depigmentation may occur. Telangiectasia may be present. Freckling and lentigo occur particularly on face and back of hands. Sweating is decreased due to dimished function of eccrine glands. Increased sensitivity to heat and cold may be apparent.

2. *Hair*: Graying begins at temples and extends to vertex of scalp, but may not occur at axilla, presternum, or pubis. Recession of scalp hair begins in males at age 20, and by age 50, one-half of male population has some baldness. Between age 40 and 70 over 60% of women also show bitemporal hairline recession. With reduction of hair follicle density, axillary hair may disappear, but rarely pubic hair. Some facial hair is normal in aging women. Leg hair becomes scanty in men and women. Eyebrows and nasal hair in men becomes longer and coarser.

3. *Nails*: Rate of nail growth decreased. This is associated with loss of luster, increasing thickness, brittleness, and flaking as well as the appearance of Beau's lines.

IV. ABNORMAL CONDITIONS

A. *Pediatric*: Eczema, head lice, impetigo, insect bites, pityriasis rosea, port wine staining, primary and secondary skin lesions, scales, strawberry hemangioma, tinea, warts.

B. *Adult*: See lesion charts, tables 3-1, 3-2, 3-3.

4
Head, Skull, Scalp, and Face

I. HISTORY QUESTIONS

A Headache?
B Trauma to head or face?
C Sinus pain?
D Scalp itching?
E Scalp bugs (infestations)?

II. CLINICAL EXAMINATION

A. *Preparation*

1. *Position*: Client in sitting position fully clothed or disrobed and draped.
2. *Equipment*: Measuring tape, stethoscope.

B. *Inspection and palpation*

1. *Head, skull, and scalp*
    a. Size? See physical growth charts, Appendix II. (NL diameter appropriate for age and body size.)
    b. Contour? (NL symmetrical—slight asymmetries of no significance (see fig. 4-1). Generally round with frontal areas prominent anteriorally and parietal-occipital areas prominent posteriorally. No separation of suture lines after age 19 months (see fig. 4-2).

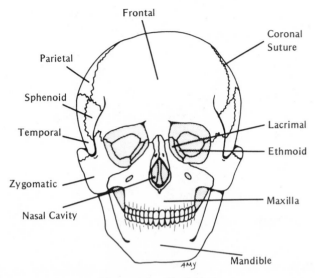

Figure 4-1 Facial bones

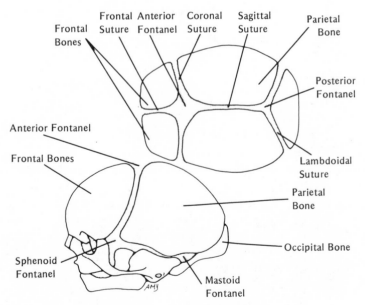

Figure 4-2 Infant skull bones

1. Head, skull, and scalp cont.

    c.   Hair color, character, density, and distribution? (NL lustrous and flexible, not brittle or dull; no patchy alopecia or thinning. Density and distribution appropriate to sex, age, and genetic heritage. Anterior and posterior hairlines not excessively low. Color and character consistent with genetic heritage.)

    d.   Position? (NL midline when relaxed. No visible tilting of head.)

    e.   Scalp hygiene? (NL no seborrhea, no lesions, no head lice or other infestations.)

    f.   Masses? (NL none.) Location? Contour? Consistency? Tenderness? Induration? Mobility? Boundaries?

2. Face

    a.   Proportions? (NL spacing and symmetry consistent with genetic heritage. Minor asymmetries of no significance. No striking enlargements of facial bones without familial precedent: no prognathism, micrognathia, frontal bossing, or hypertelorism or hypotelorism (see fig. 4-1). Top of pinna crosses eye-occiput line; angle of pinna no more than 10 degrees off vertical.)

    b.   Color, pigmentation? (NL appropriate to genetic heritage, even distribution, no areas of depigmentation, no recent change in pigmentation, no jaundice or cyanosis.)

    c.   Expression? (NL alert, not dull, sleepy, excited, anxious or masklike; expressive movement smooth and fluid.)

    d.   Movement? (NL symmetrical, able to clench teeth, move jaw side to side—Cranial Nerve V, Trigeminal; able to purse lips and wrinkle forehead—Cranial Nerve VII, facial nerve.)

    e.   Sensation? (NL intact pain, temperature and light touch sensations over temporal, maxillary, and mandibular areas of face—Cranial Nerve V, Trigeminal, see fig. 4-3.)

    f.   Edema? (NL none.)

    g.   Lesions? (NL none.)

    h.   Masses? (NL none.) Location? Size? Contour? Consistency? Tenderness? Induration? Mobility? Boundaries?

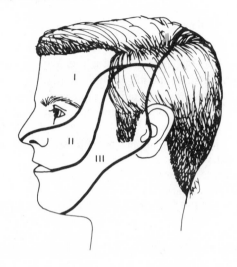

Figure 4-3   Facial sensory areas. The sensory portion of the trigeminal nerve has three divisions which are represented on the skin surface as indicated above: 1, opthalmic; 2, maxillary; 3, mandibular.

3. *Lymph nodes*: Suboccipital, preauricular and postauricular, submental (NL nonpalpable, nontender.)

    a. Size?

    b. Mobility?   *d.* Temperature?

    c. Consistency?   *e.* Tenderness?

C. *Percussion*? (NL no pain or tenderness in frontal and maxillary sinus area.)

D. *Auscultation*? (NL no cranial bruits.)

III. LIFE-CYCLE VARIATIONS IN PHYSICAL FINDINGS

A. *Developmental*: Head size changes in dimension and proportion (in reference to body) until adolescence. It reaches 90% final size by age

6. Suture lines may be overriding at birth, flatten by age 6 months, anterior fontanels close by 19 months, posterior by 4–8 weeks. Facial bones change in proportion with varying growth rates, particularly jaw and nasal bones. Newborns delivered vaginally often have soft swelling with edema and bruising of occipitoparietal region, as well as molding of the frontal and parietal bones which usually resolves in the first week of life.

B. *Degenerative*: Loss, thinning, and whitening of scalp hair. Loss of skin moisture, subcutaneous fat, and skin elasticity occurs, which leads to facial skin redundancy, prominence of orbital and facial bones, and sagging of facial features. Edentulous state is associated with jaw bone resorption, shrinkage of lower portion of face, and infolding of mouth. Loss of skin capillaries leads to graying of facial skin. Pain, as might accompany chronic skin lesions, sometimes absent due to reduction of nerve condition.

IV. ABNORMAL CONDITIONS

A. *Pediatric*: Cephalohematoma, cranial stenosis, facial asymmetries due to congenital and genetic syndromes, head lice, hydrocephalus, microcephalus, scalp infection, sinusitis.

B. *Adult*: Paget's disease, posttraumatic hematoma.

5
Eye

I. HISTORY QUESTIONS

A Ever had eyes tested? Date of last vision test? Results? Who tested?

B Wear glasses? Contact lenses? Last time glasses or contact lenses changed? What type correction?

C Difficulty seeing? Blurring vision? See double (diplopia)?

D Pain around eyes? Itching? Red eye (conjunctivitis)?

E Swollen eyelids?

F Crossed eyes (strabismus)? Eye fatigue?

G Blind spots (scotomata)?

H Excessive tearing (epiphoria)?

I Pain in eyes? Eye pain in bright light (photophobia)?

J Ever tested for glaucoma? Results?

II. CLINICAL EXAMINATION

A. *Preparation*

1. *Position*: Client in sitting position.

2. *Equipment*: Ophthalmoscope, tonometer, anesthetic drops, dilating drops, pen light, adult or pediatric vision testing chart.

B. *Inspection*

1. *External structures (see fig. 5-1)*
    a. Eyebrows and eyelashes
        1. Color and texture? (NL consistent with age and genetic heritage, no absence of pigment.)

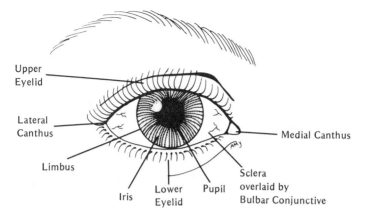

Figure 5-1   Anatomy of the external eye

2. Condition? (NL shiny, flexible hair shafts, not broken, dry; lash follicles nontender, without redness or swelling.)

3. Quantity? (NL present in moderate to dense thickness; scant density or complete absence suggests disease, genetic condition, or plucking.)

4. Distribution? (NL thick short eyebrow hairs along arched bony prominence above orbit; eyelash hairs, long or short, connect to movable edges of eyelids in double or triple rows.)

b. Eyelids

1. Color? (NL skin color appropriate to genetic heritage, no redness.)

2. Conformation? (NL consistent with genetic heritage. No entropion or ectropion. No epicanthal folds persisting beyond age 10 or Mongolian folds persisting beyond age 1 in non-Asiatic children.)

3. Position? (NL symmetrical full retraction on command—Cranial Nerve III, Oculomotor. No ptosis. No lid lag; cornea and bulbar conjunctiva not exposed on closure. No narrowing of palpebral fissure—squinting—in the absence of high light intensity.)

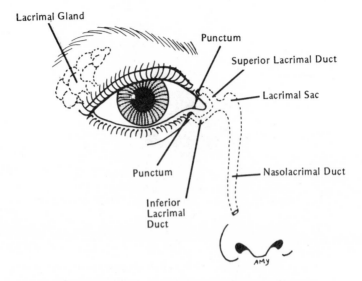

Figure 5-2   Anatomy of lacrimal apparatus

b. *Eyelids cont.*
    4. Blinking? (NL 6-12 blinks per minute. No blepharo-
        spasm or staring.)
    5. Edema? (NL none.)
    6. Lesions? (NL none.)
c. Lacrimal apparatus (see fig. 5-2).
    1. Color? (NL pink, no erythema in area of puncta or
        ducts.)
    2. Tearing? (NL no spilling of tears in absence of stimulus.
        No epiphora, no absence of tears, i.e., dysautonomia.)
    3. Swelling? (NL no distention.)
    4. Discharge? (NL none.)
d. Eyeball and orbit
    1. Eyeball size? (NL symmetrical, no microphthalmia.)
    2. Orbital contour? (NL smoothly arched. No excessive
        prominence of supraorbital ridges.)

3. Position of eyeball in socket? (NL symmetrical depth, no enophthalmos or exophthalmos.)
4. Spacing of orbits? (NL consistent with genetic heritage. No hypertelorism or hypotelorism.)

e. Conjunctiva
   1. Color? (NL transparent, palpebral conjunctiva appearing pink; bulbar, white. No pallor of palpebral conjunctiva, and no red, yellow, or brown discoloration of palpebral or bulbar conjunctiva. Small amount of injection at angles of eye of no pathological significance.)
   2. Moisture? (NL glistening, moist appearance, no dullness.)
   3. Lesions, swelling? (NL none, no cobblestoning.)

f. Sclera
   1. Color? (NL white to light brown, varying with genetic heritage. No yellow, dark blue, or pie-shaped brown discoloration.)
   2. Contour? (NL smoothly rounded, no irregularities.)

g. Cornea
   1. Color? (NL transparent, no opacities or pigmentations on oblique illumination.)
   2. Contour? (NL smoothly rounded, no abrasions, ulcerations, swellings.)
   3. Depth (anterior chamber)? (NL no shadow cast on iris on oblique illumination.)
   4. Sensitivity? (NL brisk lid closure on touching cornea with wisp of sterile cotton—Cranial Nerve V; Trigeminal.)

h. Iris
   1. Color? (NL symmetrical and consistent with genetic heritage. No pink or blue pigment, no absence or dulling of color, no white speckling, no circumferential erythematous or copper-colored rings.)
   2. Shape? (NL circumferential, smooth, slightly concave. No coloboma.)

i. Pupil
   1. Size? (NL 3–6 mm, symmetrical, neither widely dilated nor pin point in average room light; 0.5 mm difference in diameter of no pathological significance.)
   2. Shape? (NL perfectly round.)

3. Reactivity? (NL prompt constriction in response to direct and consensual light stimulus and accommodation for near vision. No sluggishness or absence of reactivity—Cranial Nerve III, oculomotor.)

j. Eye alignment: (NL corneal light reflex symmetrical.)

k. Extraocular movement: (NL smooth, symmetrical movements through all six cardinal positions of gaze—no divergence in any position. Slight nystagmus in most lateral position of no pathological significance. Cover test negative—Cranial Nerve III, Oculomotor; Cranial Nerve IV, Trochlear? Cranial Nerve VI, Abducens. (See fig. 5-3.)

2. *Internal structures*: The funduscopic examination (see fig. 5-4).

a. Lens? (NL clear, no opacities, appearance of circular red or reddish orange reflex as light shown into pupil. No trembling of iris associated with lens dislocation.)

b. Vitreous? (NL clear, no cloudiness or dark spots, appearance of red reflex as light shown into eye.)

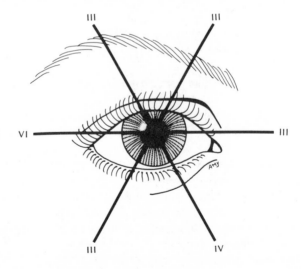

Figure 5-3 Cardinal positions of gaze. The roman numerals indicate the cranial nerve controlling gaze in that direction.

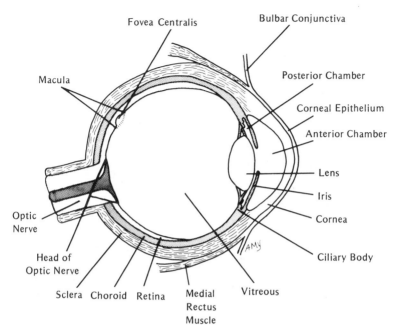

Figure 5-4 Cross section of the eye

c. Disc
   1. Size? (NL approximately 1.5 mm.)
   2. Shape? (NL round, oval.)
   3. Color? (NL pale reddish yellow to creamy pink.)
   4. Cup? (NL often present—though sometimes absent—as smooth grayish concave area, central to disc, cup to disc ratio 0.2 : 1.0.)
   5. Margins? (NL temporal margin sharp, nasal margin less defined. May be surrounded by white scleral ring.)
d. Vessels
   1. Arterioles? (NL brighter red and smaller in diameter—ratio 2 : 3—than accompanying venules, light reflection appearing as narrow light streak in center. Progress toward periphery in gentle curves—no tortuosity.)

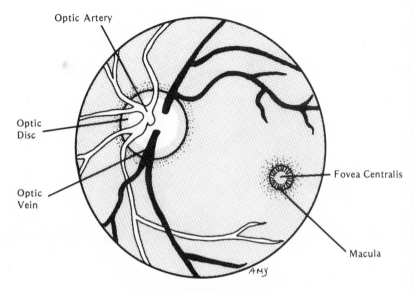

Figure 5-5 Fundus of the eye

d. vessels cont.

 2. Venules? (NL larger in diameter than arterioles—ratio
     3 : 2. Purplish red with patchy or no light reflection.
     Slightly pulsating. No venule discontinuity at arteriolar
     crossings.)

C. *Palpation*

 1. Ocular tension? (NL prompt rebound of indented sclera against
     withdrawing finger.)
 2. Ocular compressibility? (NL eyeball displaceable 0.5 cm into
     orbital fat.)

D. *Percussion*: Not part of the conventional eye examination.

E. *Auscultation?* (NL no bruits.)

F. *Vision testing*: Cranial Nerve II, Optic
 1. Visual acuity? (NL able to accurately call out letters in 20/20
     test line of Snellen chart or other eye-testing chart, from distance
     of 20 feet or 60 meters; see fig. 5-5.)

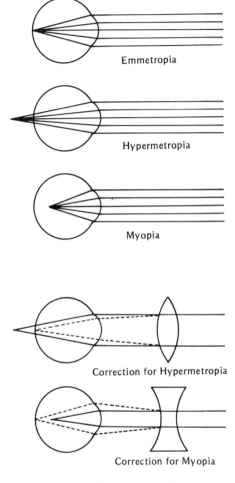

Figure 5-6   Refraction and correction

2. *Color vision?* (NL able to differentiate between green and red lines on Snellen chart.)
3. *Near vision?* (NL able to read newsprint at distance of 1 foot or 30 cm.)

F. Vision Testing cont.

    4.   *Visual field integrity?* (NL able by confrontation to identify object 60 degrees nasally, 50 degrees upward, 90 degrees temporally, and 70 degrees downward.)

G. *Tonometry:* (NL 12–22 mm Hg.)

III. LIFE-CYCLE VARIATIONS IN PHYSICAL FINDINGS

A. *Developmental:* Epicanthal folds found normally in Oriental children and 20% of Caucasian children, disappear by 10 years of age. Tearing not common before 3 months of age. Sclera slightly bluish in newborns, and small conjunctiva and scleral hemorrhages may appear in the absence of significant pathology. Pupils of infants are slightly smaller in size. In sighted newborns head dorsiflexion and eye blinking are responses to bright light (optic blink reflex), as are direct and consensual pupillary responses. Visual activity at age 3 is approximately 20/40; at age 4, 20/30; at age 6 to 7, 20/20. Intermittent convergent horizontal strabismus may be seen normally prior to 3 months of age. Divergent strabismus is abnormal. Short periods of nystagmus may be seen in an infant who is not yet focusing.

B. *Degenerative:* Gradual loss of lid elasticity leads to drooping of eyelids (blepharochalasis). Pupils normally slightly smaller in aged. Senile plaques and degenerative infiltrates occasionally found on conjunctiva. Degenerative material may appear within limbus of cornea (arcus senilis). Lens may show loss of transparency which leads to clouding of vision, and vitreous floaters and retinal exudates may appear. Choroidal sclerosis and macular degeneration may be found on funduscopic examination. Some loss of visual acuity and accommodation usually occurs with aging, as well as decrease in extent of visual field, speed of dark adaptation, and sensitivity to blue hues.

IV. ABNORMAL CONDITIONS

A. *Pediatric:* Chalazia, conjunctivitis, color blindness, hordeola, myopia, ptosis of the lid, strabismus.

B. *Adult:* Cataracts, chalazia, conjunctivitis, detached retina, ectropion and entropion, glaucoma, hordeola, occulsion of retinal vessels, presbyopia, pterygia.

6
Ear

I. HISTORY QUESTIONS

A Ear infection? How often?
B Draining ears (discharge)? How often? Pus (purulent discharge)? Clear? Color?
C Ear trauma? When? Describe.
D Ear pain? How often? Pull at ears?
E Buzzing (tinnitus) or other noises in ears?
F Dizziness, vertigo, or nausea associated with hearing difficulty?
G Poor hearing? Noticed when?
H Bothered by noise (hearing sensitivity)?
I Certain types of noise bother more than others (recruitment)?
J Difficulty understanding others (speech discrimination)?
K Speech problem?

II. CLINICAL EXAMINATION

A. *Preparation*

1. *Position*: Client in sitting position, head tilted away from examiner. Small child should sit in adult's lap. Infant supine on examining table with arms elevated and restrained next to head, head turned.

2. *Equipment*: Watch, tuning fork (256, 512, 1024 cps), otoscope.

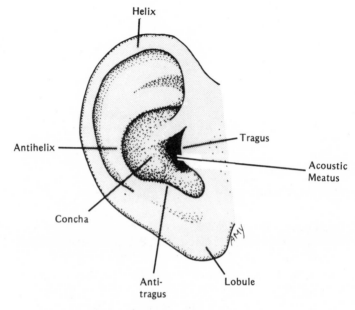

Figure 6-1   Anatomy of the external ear

B. *Inspection and palpation*

1. *Pinna* (see fig. 6-1)
   a. Size? (NL no microtia less than 4 cm in vertical span or macrotia, greater than 10 cm in vertical span.)
   b. Shape? (NL no gnarling or thickening.)
   c. Position? (NL top of pinna crosses eye-occiput line, pinna no more than 10 degrees off vertical line; bilateral symmetrical placement.)
   d. Trophi? (NL none.)
   e. Darwinian tubercle? (NL none.)
   f. Lesions? (NL none.)
   g. Masses? (NL none.) Location? Size? Contour? Consistency? Tenderness? Induration? Mobility? Boundaries?
   h. Tragal tenderness? (NL none.)
2. *Mastoid*: (NL no swelling, redness or tenderness.)

3. *Auditory canal* (see fig. 6-2)
    a. Formation? (NL no atresia.)
    b. Cerumen? (NL small lobules, yellow to brown color, consistency of petroleum jelly, appearing oily, not dull or crusty, not blocking ear canal.)
    c. Foreign objects? (NL none.)
    d. Inflammation, tenderness? (NL none.)
    e. Lesions? Nodules? Cysts? Polyps? Scaling? (NL none.)

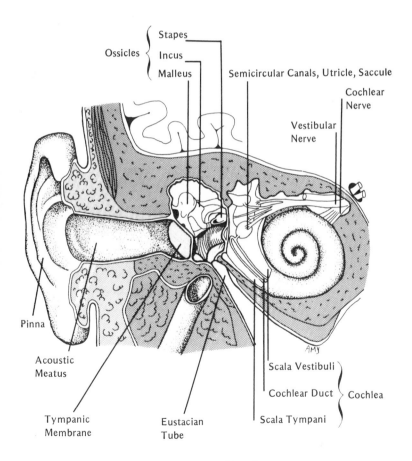

Figure 6-2   Anatomy of hearing apparatus

4. *Tympanic membrane*: The Otoscopic Examination.

    a. Color? (NL translucent, shiny, pearly gray membrane, not amber, blue white, pink or red.)

    b. Position? (NL oblique relative to ear canal, superior-posterior portion closest to orifice, anterior-inferior portion farthest away. Not retracted or bulging.)

    c. Landmarks? (NL manubrium, short process, umbo, anterior and posterior malleolar folds visible, but not exaggerated. Annulus white and dense appearing, no perforations. Light reflex present and intact in the anterior-inferior quadrant. See fig. 6-3.)

    d. Mobility? (NL drum bulges outward in response to increased pressure transmitted up eustacian tube when client blows against closed lips with nostrils pinched.)

    e. Fluid level? (NL none.)

    f. Air bubbles? (NL none.)

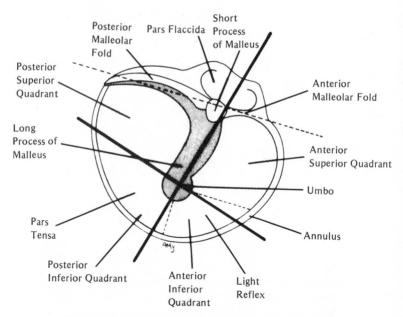

Figure 6-3   Tympanic membrane and landmarks

C. ***Percussion and ausculation***: Not part of the conventional ear examination.

D. ***Hearing testing***: Cranial Nerve VIII, Acoustic, cochlear branch.
1. *Voice test*: (NL with opposite ear masked, client hears examiner whisper from 2 feet and repeats words whispered.)
2. *Watch tick test*: (NL with opposite ear masked, client to hear watch tick from same distance at which examiner just able to hear it.)
3. *Tuning fork tests*
    a. Weber: (NL client hears tuning fork equally loud with both ears. In conductive loss sound lateralizes to poor ear. In sensorineural loss sound lateralizes to good ear.)
    b. Rinne: (NL client hears tuning fork twice as long by air conduction as by bone conduction. In mild conductive loss hear sound longer by air conduction but not twice as long. In moderate conductive loss, hears sound equally long by both means. In severe conductive loss, hears sound longer by bone than air. In sensorineural loss, hears sound longer by air but perception reduced by both modes.)
    c. Schwabach: (NL client and examiner cease hearing tuning fork at same time. In conductive loss client hears sound longer than examiner. In sensorineural loss examiner hears sound longer than client.)
4. *Pure-tone audiometry*: (NL hears sound in all frequencies at 0–20 decibels.)

III. LIFE-CYCLE VARIATIONS IN PHYSICAL FINDINGS

A. ***Developmental***: Hearing acute in early infancy as manifested by alertness to noise stimuli. A brisk Moro response should follow loud sudden noises. Hearing newborns blink in response to loud noises (acoustic blink reflex). The head turns toward the source of sound by 3 to 4 months of age. In childhood, hearing is manifested by normal responses to tuning fork tests and audiometry. It is also manifested by attentive, responsive behavior and normal progression in social and educational spheres. Speech development reflects hearing acuteness in childhood, and by the 7th year all sounds should be phonetically correct. Pinna grows proportionate to head. Obliqueness of tympanic membrane is more pronounced in children. Auditory canal curves upward in young children and downward in older children and adults.

B. *Degenerative*: Gradual sensorineural hearing loss accompanies aging. Threshold for all pure-tone frequencies increases, but high-tone thresholds (4000 cps) increases more. Speech reception and discrimination may be affected. Auditory reaction time increases after 70 years of age. Loss of elasticity of the pinna leads to elongation of lobe which averages 12 mm by age 80. Accompanying this is wrinkling of the lobe in a linear oblique pattern. Frequently dense white plaques visualized on tympanic membrane are manifestations of past infection. The aged drum characteristically appears thicker, whiter, more opaque and often shows a loss of luster.

IV. ABNORMAL CONDITIONS

A. *Pediatric*: Atresia of auditory canal, cholesteotoma, congenital deafness, foreign body, impacted cerumen, membrane perforation, otitis externa, otitis media, ototoxic deafness, postmeningitic deafness.

B. *Adult*: Acoustic neuroma, cholesteotoma, impacted cerumen, Ménière's syndrome, malignant lesions of external ear, otosclerosis, tympanic membrane perforations.

7
Nose, Mouth, and Throat

I. HISTORY QUESTIONS

A   Runny nose (rhinorrhea)? Continuous (chronic)?

B   Bloody nose (epistaxis)?

C   Broken nose?

D   Hay fever (seasonal rhinitis)?

E   Colds (URI)? How often?

F   Can't breathe through nose (nasal obstruction)?

G   Snore?

H   Change in sense of smell?

I   Use toothbrush and dental floss regularly (oral hygiene)?

J   Had fluoride treatment?

K   Date last dental examination?

L   Wear dentures?

M   Toothache? Tooth sensitivity? Any problems with teeth? Loss of teeth?

N   Sore mouth? Sore tongue? Sore gums? Sore jaw? Sore throat?

O   Grind teeth (bruxism)?

P   Bleeding gums?

Q   Change in sense of taste?

R   Voice changes? Persistent hoarseness?

S   Difficulty swallowing?

T   Frequent throat infections?

II. CLINICAL EXAMINATION

A. *Preparation*

   1.   *Position*: Client in comfortable sitting position. Infant supine, arms extended and restrained next to head. Young child in adult's lap.

   2.   *Equipment*: Nasal speculum, pen light, tongue blade, and gloves.

B. *Inspection*

1. *Nasal cavity*: The speculum examination
   a. Turbinates? (NL no swelling, middle turbinate clearly visible on lateral wall. No polyps or other lesions.)
   b. Septum? (NL evenly divides nasal cavity into two equal chambers. Transillumination of septum produces pink light; no tumor or perforation of septum. Septal deviation not obstructing airway of no significance. Small spurs or ridges of no significance.)
   c. Mucosa? (NL pink, not fiery red or pale grayish. Smooth and moist appearing, no crusting, edema, or lesions. Covered with clear mucus.)
2. *Mouth and pharynx*
   a. Lips
      1. Shape? (NL symmetrical, consistent with genetic heritage, no incomplete fusion.)
      2. Position? (NL symmetrical placement when teeth clenched with lips open—Cranial Nerve VII, Facial.)
      3. Movement? (NL symmetrical for all facial expressions.)
      4. Condition? (NL no cracks or fissures, no cheilosis.)
      5. Color? (NL pink to brown, no cyanosis, no pallor.)
      6. Lesions? (NL none.)
   b. Oral cavity and palate
      1. Teeth: (NL 32 present in good repair, no untreated caries, no malocclusion, dentures well fitted.)
      2. Gums? (NL pink, moist, not retracted, inflamed, bleeding, or discolored.)
      3. Tongue
         a. Color? (NL similar to oral mucosa; not red or beefy looking.)
         b. Texture? (NL irregular—taste buds apparent, no denuding or smooth appearance. "Coated," "hairy," or geographic tongue of no pathologic significance. Inferior surface: small with easily visible venous pattern.)
         c. Size? (NL fits easily into mouth, no deep furrowing.)

        d.   Movement? (NL protrudes in midline, no tremors—
             Cranial Nerve XII: Hypoglossal.)

        e.   Lesions? (NL none.)

   4. Sublinguinal veins: (NL not varicose.)

   5. Frenulum: (NL able to protrude tongue between teeth.)

   6. Buccal mucosa

        a.   Color? (NL pink, no plaques or hemiangiomas.)

        b.   Texture? (NL smooth, moist, shiny.)

        c.   Lesions? (NL none.)

   7. Parotid duct: (NL patent orifice large enough to accept
      probe readily; pressure over duct opening yields clear
      secretion.)

   8. Submaxillary gland: (NL patent orifices next to frenu-
      lum, producing clear secretions when expressed.)

   9. Palate

        a.   Color? (NL soft palate pink, hard palate whiter.)

        b.   Contour? (NL gently, smoothly, symmetrically
             arched. No high or pointed arch. No visible cleft.)

        c.   Movement? (NL palate elevates symmetrically,
             uvula rises at midline—Cranial Nerve IX, Glosso-
             pharyngeal, and Cranial Nerve X, Vagus.)

        d.   Lesions? (NL none.)

 10. Uvula

        a.   Length? (NL free margin should not obstruct oral
             pharynx.)

        b.   Structure? (NL free-hanging, single, pear-shaped
             projection. Bifid uvula may be normal but is occa-
             sionally associated with submucous cleft palate.)

        c.   Lesions? (NL none.)

 c. Pharynx

   1. Tonsils

        a.   Size? (NL present, symmetrical, not projected be-
             yond tonsillar pillar, no swelling.)
             (*Note*: Evaluation scale for recording tonsil size: 1+
             tonsil edges only seen; 2+ tonsil edges midway be-
             tween pillars and uvula; 3+ tonsil edges touching
             uvula; 4+ tonsil edges meet midline.)

        b.   Color? (NL same as oral mucosa.)

        c.   Contour? (NL irregular, smoothly rolling surface, sometimes with shallow crypts which may collect debris appearing as white spots.)

        d.   Membrane? (NL none.)

        e.   Lesions? (NL none.)

    2.   Posterior pharyngeal wall

        a.   Color? (NL pink; small amount injection or hyperemia not significant. Covered with clear mucus.)

        b.   Movement? (NL intact gag reflex, with midline elevation of uvula, able to swallow—Cranial Nerve IX, Glossopharyngeal, and Cranial Nerve X, Vagus.)

        c.   Edema? (NL none.)

        d.   Discharge? (NL none.)

        e.   Lesions? (NL none. Small red or pink spots are normal dots of lymphoid tissue.)

C.   *Palpation*: The bimanual examination

    1.   *Mouth*

        a.   Floor? (NL nontender, no swellings, masses, plaques, lesions.)

        b.   Walls? (NL soft, compressible, nontender, no lesions, tumors, plaques.)

        c.   Soft palate? (NL no submucous cleft.)

        d.   Salivary ducts? (NL nontender, no calculi.)

    2.   *Tongue*? (NL soft, uniformly compressible, nontender tissue. No swelling or masses.)

    3.   *Frontal and maxillary sinuses*? (NL nontender.)

D.   *Percussion*: Frontal and maxillary sinuses? (NL nontender.)

E.   *Auscultation*: Not part of the conventional nose, mouth, and throat examination.

F.   *Assessment of taste, smell, and voice*

    1.   *Smell*? (NL with eyes closed able to differentiate familiar odors—Cranial Nerve I, Olfactory.)

    2.   *Taste*? (NL can differentiate samples of sweet, sour, bitter, and salty tastes—Cranial Nerve VII, Facial, and Cranial Nerve IX, Glossopharyngeal.)

3. Voice: (NL pitch consistent with sex and genetic heritage. No hoarseness—Cranial Nerve X, Vagus.)

III. LIFE-CYCLE VARIATIONS IN PHYSICAL FINDINGS

A. Developmental: The mouth of a newborn is edentulous, but may show small cysts on gum ridges which disappear in 4 to 8 weeks. Little saliva is produced in the first 3 months of life. Deciduous teeth erupt at approximately 6 months of age, beginning with lower incisors. All 20 are present by age 2½ years. Permanent teeth begin to appear around the 6th year, with the final third molars coming in between ages 17 and 25. Until puberty tonsils may be 2+ enlarged in the absence of pathology, and then will gradually shrink behind tonsillar pillars. Male voice lowers in pitch at puberty, and nasal and jaw bones grow at an accelerated rate during this period.

B. Degenerative: Teeth become increasingly worn and are lost due to the aging process and poor care. Marked shrinkage of the lower face may occur, with infolding of the mouth. Nose elongates slightly with age, and some loss occurs in the acuity of the sense of smell. Taste buds may appear atrophic, and some deterioration of taste discrimination may occur. Voice pitch sometimes lowers in postmenopausal females.

IV. ABNORMAL CONDITIONS

A. Pediatric: Allergic rhinitis, bite defects, URI, congenital lip and palate defects, dental caries, herpes simplex, epistaxis, obstruction from foreign objects, tonsillitis, trauma.

B. Adult: Allergic rhinitis, cancer of larynx, colds, denture lesions, deviated nasal septum, epistaxis, leukoplakia, nasal basal cell carcinoma, oral cancer, sinus malignancies.

8
Neck

I. HISTORY QUESTIONS

A Stiffness?
B Pain?
C Lumps (masses)?

II. CLINICAL EXAMINATION

A. *Preparation*

1. *Position*: Client in sitting position. Head rotated to side opposite of that being examined.
2. *Equipment*: Stethoscope.

B. *Inspection*

1. *Structures visualized*: Sternocleidomastoid muscle, jugular veins, thyroid cartilage, trachea, clavicle, carotid pulsations.
2. *Symmetry*? (NL symmetrical, nonwebbed appearance, angles of the jaw equidistant from respective shoulders.)
3. *Neck curvature*? (NL cervical concavity.)
4. *Head movement*? (NL smooth and coordinated, no tics or spasms.)
5. *Range of motion*
   a. Flexion? (NL 45 degrees, able to touch chin to sternum.)
   b. Extension? (NL 55 degrees.)

      c.   Lateral bending? (NL 40 degrees.)

      d.   Rotation? (NL 70 degrees–Cranial Nerve XI, Accessory.)

  6. *Pulsation?* (NL in supine position visible at base of neck, diffuse and undulent, augmented on expiration, diminished on inspiration.)

  7. Venous distension? (NL neck veins flat at 45 degrees or higher sitting position.)

  8. Thyroid enlargement? (NL none.)

  9. Lymphadenopathy? (NL none.)

 10. Masses, swelling, scars, skin discolorations? (NL none.)

C. *Palpation*

  1. *Lymph nodes*–posterior cervical, anterior cervical, submental, submandibular: (NL non-palpable, nontender, small posterior nodes of no pathological significance.) Size? Mobility? Temperature? Tenderness? Consistency? (See fig. 8-1.)

  2. *Thyroid:* (NL soft, barely palpable, no nodules, estimated weight of 25 gms.) (See fig. 8-2.)

  3. *Trachea?* (NL midline at suprasternal notch.)

  4. *Pulsations?* Carotid arteries? (NL amplitude symmetrical, prompt smooth upstroke 0.01-second duration, descending limb more gradual. Caution: Simultaneous bilateral palpation of carotids should not be done.)

  5. *Masses?* (NL none.) Tenderness? Location? Size? Contour? Induration? Mobility? Boundaries?

D. *Percussion:* Not part of the conventional neck examination.

E. *Auscultation*

  1. *Carotid bruits?* (NL none.) Subclavian? (NL none.) Thyroid gland? (NL none.)

  2. *Murmurs?* (NL none.)

  3. *Venous hum?* (Presence usually of no significance.)

F. *Assessment of muscle strength?* (NL able to rotate, flex, and hyperextend neck against resistance.)

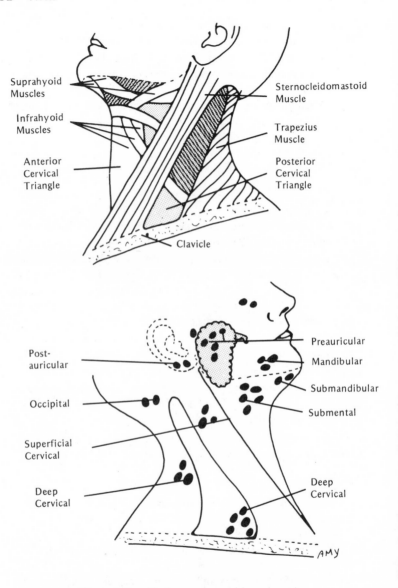

Figure 8-1   Neck muscles and lymph nodes

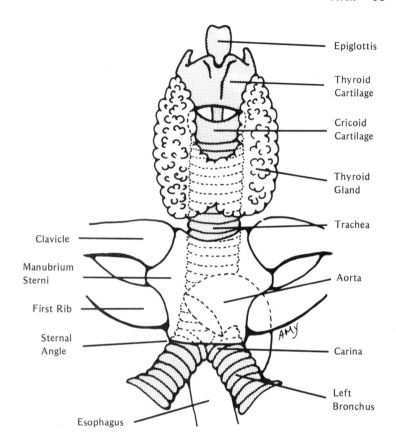

Figure 8-2   Internal anatomy of the neck

III. LIFE-CYCLE VARIATIONS IN PHYSICAL FINDINGS

A. *Developmental*: Neck diameter and length small in relationship to head size in infancy and early childhood. Gradual increase in proportionate size of neck with growth of torso. Head control evident beginning at 3 months of age and stable at 5 months of age.

B. *Degenerative*: Loss of range of motion occurs with vertebral joint degeneration. Loss of muscle tone and skin elasticity leads to more evident appearance of neck arteries and veins. Reduced neck muscle mass and strength are associated with weakening of head movement against resistance. Shortening of the neck from vertebral column shrinkage causes a descent of thyroid lobes in relation to the clavicle.

IV. ABNORMAL CONDITIONS

A. *Pediatric*: Cervical lymphadenopathy due to systemic and local conditions, torticollis.

B. *Adult*: Ankylosing spondylitis, carotid atherosclerosis, cervical osteo-arthritis, hyperthyroidism, hypothyroidism, malignancies, thyroid tumor.

9
Breasts and Axillae

I. HISTORY QUESTIONS

A   Breast self-exam? How often?
B   Breast lumps (masses)? Where? Date noticed? Relation to period (menses)?
C   Breast tenderness? Where? Date noticed? Relation to period (menses)?
D   Any discharge from breasts? Color? Amount? Consistency? Odor? Date noticed?
E   Any swelling of breasts? Recent change in bra size? Relation to period (menses)? Pregnancy? Breast feeding (lactating)?
F   Any axillary tenderness? Lumps? Where? Date noticed? Relation to period menses?
G   Any rash? Occur with deodorant?

II. CLINICAL EXAMINATION

A. *Preparation*

1. *Position*: Client disrobed to waist, breasts draped, sitting and lying with hands on hips, chest muscles tensed, and hands overhead.
2. *Equipment*: None.

B. *Inspection*

1. *Breasts*
   a. Size? (NL 2nd or 3rd rib to 6th or 7th costal cartilage, edge of sternum to anterior axillary line, estimated weight 150–200 gms.)
   b. Symmetry? (NL symmetrical to slightly asymmetrical, considering no recent change.)
   c. Contour? (NL no skin retraction, dimpling, flattening, masses.) (See fig. 9-1.)
   d. Color? (NL even distribution of pigment and consistent with genetic heritage and remainder of body.)
   e. Hair pattern? (NL female—none to sparse, hair away from midline of no significance; male—none to heavy.)
   f. Venous pattern? (NL not prominent.)
   g. Skin appearance? (NL not tight or shiny.)
   h. Edema? (NL none—no pronounced hair follicles or follicular openings, no "orange peel" or "pig skin" appearance.) (See fig. 9-1.)
   i. Lesions? Scars? Masses? (NL none.) Location?
   j. Rashes? Ulcerations? (NL none.) Date first noticed? Drainage? Odor? Consistency? Amount? Color? Crusting? Size? Location?

2. *Areola*
   a. Shape? (NL round.)
   b. Color? (NL same as nipple.)
   c. Hair? (NL sparse, circumferential to areola.)
   d. Retraction? (NL none.)
   e. Masses? (NL small elevations not pathologically significant.)

3. *Nipple*
   a. Size? Shape? (NL round.) Inverted? (Significant only if recent or unilateral.)
   b. Symmetry? (NL slight asymmetry.)
   c. Color? (NL darker pigment than breast skin.)
   d. Distance between nipples?
      (*Note*: Apparent wide setting of nipples in the absence of breast development may indicate genetic disease.)

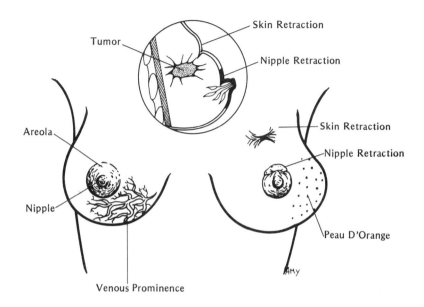

Figure 9-1   Abnormalities of the breast

    e.   Retraction? (NL none.) (See fig. 9-1.)

    f.   Rashes? Ulcerations? (NL none.) Date noticed? Drainage? Odor? Consistency? Amount? Color? Crusting? Size? Location?

4. *Axillae*

    a.   Hair distribution? (NL present.)

    b.   Cleanliness? Body odor?

    c.   Discoloration? (NL none.)

    d.   Bulging? Retraction? Edema? (NL none.)

    e.   Enlarged lymph nodes or masses? (NL none.)

    f.   Rashes? (NL none.) Date first noticed?

    g.   Ulcerations? (NL none.) Drainage? Amount? Color? Odor? Consistency? Size? Location?

C. *Palpation*

1. *Breasts*
   a. Consistency? (NL firm, elastic, and lobular in female; firm in male.)
   b. Premenstrual changes? (NL enlarged, tender nodes.)
   c. Masses? (NL none.) Location? Size? Contour? Consistency? Tenderness? Induration? Mobility? Boundaries?

2. *Areola*
   a. Tenderness? (NL none.)
   b. Masses? (NL none.) Location? Size? Contour? Consistency? Tenderness? Induration? Mobility? Boundaries?

3. *Nipple*
   a. Discharge? (NL none.) Color? Amount? Odor? Consistency?
   b. Tenderness? (NL none.)

4. *Axillae*
   a. Tenderness? (NL none.)
   b. Masses? (NL none.) Location? Size? Contour? Consistency? Tenderness? Induration? Mobility? Boundaries?
   c. Lymph nodes? (NL nonpalpable.)

D. *Percussion and ausculation*: Not part of the conventional breast examination.

III. LIFE-CYCLE VARIATIONS IN PHYSICAL FINDINGS

A. *Developmental*: Areolar swelling occurs in neonates due to transplacental hormones. In the young child nipples and areola grow in proportion to chest size. No budding or breast swelling apparent before age 9 in female, generally remaining flat in male. Breast budding may proceed unilaterally.

B. *Pregnancy and Lactation*: Breasts firm, hard, enlarged, lobules more distinct, vascular prominence and tenderness may be present. Clear nipple discharge last trimester.

C. *Degenerative*: Loss of tissue elasticity causes a "fried egg" appearance—flattening and dropping. Loss of subcutaneous fat with wrinkling of breast skin. Stringy feel on palpation and occasional nodularity may be sensed. Loss of axillary hair occurs, hair becoming thinner and whiter. Greater concavity of axilla results from loss of subcutaneous fat.

IV. ABNORMAL CONDITIONS

A. *Pediatric*: Supernumerary nipples, tumors, Turner's syndrome.

B. *Adult*: Adenofibroma, benign and malignant tumors, blocked mammary gland in lactation, cystic mastitis, gynocomastia, Paget's disease, traumatic fat necrosis.

10
Chest

I. HISTORY QUESTIONS

A Last Chest X ray? Date? Result?

B Cough? Often (frequency)? Dry (nature)? Spit phlegm (productive cough)? Amount? Color? Thick (viscosity)? Blood (hemoptysis)? Constant? Streaks? Clots? Frank blood? Sputum frothy? Odor? Cough up phlegm in daytime? Nighttime? When change position?

C Recent change in voice? Hoarseness?

D Ever told have emphysema? By whom?

E Short of breath (dyspnea)? Constant or come and go (intermittent)? Relation to exercise, walking, climbing stairs, or other physical effort? Rapid breathing (tachypnea)?

F Wheeze? Asthmatic attacks? Related to season, foods, animals, dust, plants, emotion?

G Chest pain? Where (location)? How bad (severity)? When started (onset)? Pain goes where (radiation)? Worsen with deep breath? Tightness in chest?

H Recent history of pneumonia?

I Night sweats?

J Contact with TB?

K Frequent colds? Bronchitis? Croup?

L Smoke? What? How much? Live with smoker?

II. CLINICAL EXAMINATION

A. *Preparation*

1. *Position*: Client sitting disrobed to waist. Young child on adult's lap, head maintained in face-front central position.
2. *Equipment*: Stethoscope with diaphragm, watch with a second hand, quiet room.

B. *Inspection*

1. *Chest* (See fig. 10-1, pp. 62-63.)
   a. Contour? (NL slightly convex with no sternal depression, funnel chest, pigeon breast, barrel chest, localized bulges, kyphosis, scoliosis, gibbus. Slight asymmetries of no pathological significance.)
   b. Dimensions? (NL anterioposterior diameter less than transverse ratio [thoracic index] 1 : 2 to 5 : 7, depending on body build.)
   c. Rib angle? (NL costal-spinal angle 45 degrees at end-expiration. Costal-zyphoid angle slightly less than 90 degrees widening with inspiration.)
   d. Contour of intercostal spaces? (NL flat or depressed, no bulging or retractions.)
   e. Movement? (NL symmetrical.)
   f. Cartilage condition? (NL no hypertrophy.)

2. *Skin*
   a. Color? (NL with exception of slightly darker areola and nipple, even distribution of pigment consistent with genetic heritage. No pallor, cyanosis, or pigment changes, no spider nevi.)
   b. Moisture? (NL warm and dry.)
   c. Scars?

3. *Respiration*
   a. Rate? (NL 12-20.)
   b. Rhythm? (NL regular cycles, with inspiratory phase slightly longer than expiratory phase.)

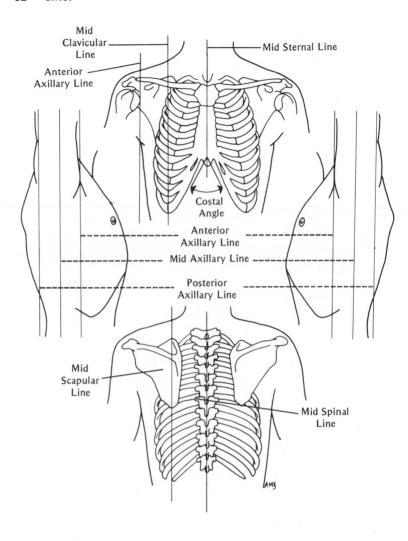

Figure 10-1   Topographical landmarks of the chest

3. *Respiration cont.*

  c. Depth? (NL even, with occasional signs, appropriate to activity.)

  d. Ratio respiratory rate to heart rate? (NL 1 : 4.)

  e. Quality of respiration? (NL quiet at rest, nonlabored. No flaring of nostrils, no subclavicular, intercostal, or abdominal retractions. No tachyphea, hyperpnea, stertorous or ataxic respirations.)

  f. Type of breathing? (NL diaphragmatic in male, costal in female; no Cheyne-Stokes, Kussmaul, or apneustic breathing patterns.)

C. *Palpation*

  1. *Tracheal alignment?* (NL equidistant from each clavicle.)

  2. *Skin temperature?* (NL same as rest of body.)

  3. *Respiratory excursion?* (NL symmetrical, 5 to 8 cm at maximal inspiration.)

  4. *Fremitus*

  a. Vocal? (NL present. Greatest intensity at anterior and posterior base of neck and along trachea and large bronchi. Least intensity over lung bases and scapulae.)

  b. Pleural friction? (NL none.)

  c. Tussive? (NL none.)

  5. *Crepitation/subcutaneous emphysema?* (NL none.)

  6. *Masses/swelling?* (NL none.)

  7. *Tenderness?* (NL none.)

D. *Percussion* (See fig. 10-2.)

  1. *Posterior chest wall*

  a. Lung borders? (NL resonance from 1st ICS to 9th ICS at end-expiration and 11th ICS at peak inspiration on left, with cardiac dullness medial to midscapular line at 5th ICS; on right, liver dullness heard at 4th-5th ICS.)

     b.   Diaphragmatic excursion? (NL dullness in the transverse diameter underlying lung resonance, varying in level with phase of respiration from 3–6 cm. Often slightly higher on right.)

  2. *Anterior chest wall*
     a.   Right lung border? (NL resonance at supraclavicular fossa extending to 5th ICS at midclavicular line and 7th ICS at midaxillary line with sternal flatness beginning at right sternal border.)
     b.   Left lung border? (NL resonance at supraclavicular fossa extending to 3rd ICS at left sternal line, to 5th ICS at or medial to midclavicular line, and 7th ICS at midaxillary line with sternal flatness beginning at left sternal border.)

E. *Auscultation*

  1. *Breath sounds*
     a.   Normal
        1. Vesicular? (NL heard over most of lung except where bronchial and bronchovesicular normally heard. Abnormal when absent over areas where expected to be heard.)
        2. Bronchial? (NL heard anterior midline over trachea; elsewhere over lung fields, associated with consolidation.)
        3. Bronchovesicular? (NL heard over upper anterior chest in 2nd ICS bilaterally, at apex of right lung, and interscapular area; elsewhere associated with consolidation.)
     b.   Adventitious: (NL no rales, rhonchi, wheezes, pleural friction rubs, or stridor.)
        1. Location?
        2. Affected by coughing?
        3. Vary with phase of respiration?
     c.   Voice sounds
        1. Vocal resonance? (NL heard as murmur through chest wall while client speaks. Absence abnormal.)

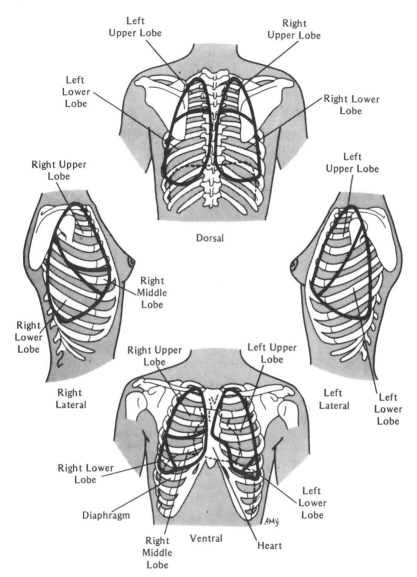

Figure 10-2   Surface projections of lung lobes.

2. Bronchophony? (NL none. Presence associated with consolidation.)
3. Whispered pectoriloquy? (NL none. Presence associated with consolidation.)
4. Egophony? (NL none. Presence associated with consolidation.)

III. LIFE-CYCLE VARIATIONS IN PHYSICAL FINDINGS

A. *Developmental*: Chest maintains a cylindrical shape through early infancy, with a thoracic index of 1. By age 1 the transverse diameter is greater and the thoracic index is 1.25, finally reaching 1.35 by age 6 and remaining stable. Chest circumference increases from 33 cm at birth to 44.6 cm at age 5 years. Respiratory rate decreases from 30 per minute at birth, to 25 per minute at 2 years, to 18 per minute at 10 years. (See normal respiratory rates for various ages, Appendix VI.) Because of the A-P diameter, hyperresonance is the normal percussion note heard over lung fields from infancy through early childhood. Breath sounds over lung fields in early childhood are bronchovesicular in nature due to the proximity of airways to the thin chest wall. Fine inspiratory rales are common and in the absence of other findings not abnormal immediately after birth and probably represent the opening of unexpanded alveoli.

B. *Degenerative*: Beginning in the 5th decade there is a senile kyphosis from an expanding anterio-posterior diameter and a shrinking of the vertical span of the thoracic spine. This together with calcification of the costal cartilage leads to reduced mobility of the ribs and loss of chest wall compliance and expansibility, often associated with partial contraction of the muscles of inspiration. Because of the expanded A-P diameter (resulting from increased lung inflation that occurs with the loss of chest wall propulsive force) the percussion note, even in the absence of disease, is hyperresonant, with a decreased intensity of breath sounds.

IV. ABNORMAL CONDITIONS

A. *Pediatric*: Asthma, croup, cystic fibrosis, foreign bodies, hyaline membrane disease, pneumonia, URI.

B. *Adult*: ARDS, asthma, atelectasis, benign tumors, bronchitis, emphysema, malignant tumors, pleural effusion, pneumonia, TB, URI.

11
Heart and Cardiovascular System

I. HISTORY QUESTIONS

A. High blood pressure (hypertension)? Symptoms?

B. Dizzy spells, vertigo? On medication?

C. Pain or tightness in chest (angina)? Relieved by nitroglycerin? How many? When started (onset)? Where started (location)? Where does pain go (radiation)? Relation to exercise, walking, climbing stairs, or other physical effort (exertion) or feeling tired (fatigue or emotional upset)? Associated symptoms such as sweating (diaphoresis), shortness of breath (dyspnea), skipping beats (palpitations), racing heart (tachycardia), or nausea?

D. Short of breath (dyspnea)? Constant or come and go (intermittent)? Produced by physical effort? Come on unexpectedly (paroxysmal)? Occur when lying down (recumbent)? Occur suddenly at night (paroxysmal nocturnal dyspnea)?

E. Able to keep up with others of own age? Able to eat or nurse without tiring? Sweat during eating?

F. How many pillows used when lying down (orthopnea)?

G. Facial skin ever appear bluish (cyanosis) or ashen (pallor)?

H. Cough? Dry? Spit mucus (productive)? What does it look like? daytime (diurnal)? Nighttime (nocturnal)? Spit blood (hemoptysis)?

I. Shoes tight at end of day (edema)? How much swelling (extent, degree)? Where? Disappear with rest?

J. Thumping or racing heart (palpitations)? Aware of sudden high heart rate (paroxysmal tachycardia) or change in regularity (dysrhythmia)? Occurs with what (association)? Lasts how long?

K. Leg pain? Occur with exercise (claudication)? Leg pain at rest (rest pain)? Change in leg color (cyanosis, pigmentation)?
L. Swollen leg veins (varicosities)?
M. Redness on leg? Area hot? Area painful?
N. Numbness or tingling of feet (paresthesia)?
O. Painful hands? One hand ever colder or warmer than other? Color different?

II. CLINICAL EXAMINATION

A. *Preparation*

1. *Position*: client in sitting and supine positions disrobed to waist.
2. *Equipment*: Stethoscope with bell and diaphragm, sphygmomanometer, watch with a second hand.

B. *Inspection*

1. *Chest contour?* (NL slightly convex with no sternal depression, funnel chest, pigeon breast, barrel chest, localized bulges, kyphosis, scoliosis, or gibbus. Slight asymmetries of no pathological significance.)

2. *Precordium* (see fig. 11-1)
   a. Bulging? Retraction? Pulsations? (NL none.)
   b. Cardiac impulse
      1. Force? (NL slight retraction, no lift or heave.)
      2. Position? (NL 5th interspace, medial to L midclavicular line.)
      3. Localization? (NL 2 cm or less in diameter.)
      4. Regularity? (NL regular, 60-100 beats per minute resting heart rate.)

3. *Neck*
   a. Venous pulsations: (NL visible at base of neck, diffuse and undulent.)
      1. Vary with respiration? (NL pulsations slightly diminished on inspiration and augmented on expiration.)

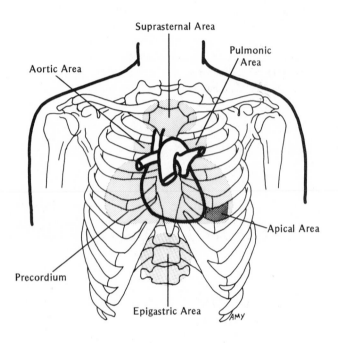

Figure 11-1   Orientation of the heart and auscultatory areas

  a.   Venous pulsations cont.
    2.   Vary with body position? (NL flat at 45-degree or higher sitting position.)
  b.   Venous distension: (NL neck veins flat at 45 degrees or higher sitting position.)
  c.   Arterial pulsations: (NL visible on extended, thin neck, no head bobbing.)

4.   *Extremities*
  a.   Hands and feet
    1.   Nail shape, color? (NL no clubbing or thickening, pale pink color.)

2. Skin color? (NL even distribution of pigment appropriate to genetic heritage and remainder of body, no cyanosis, pallor, or mottling.)

3. Hair distribution? (NL sparse to dense on proximal phalanyx in male, sparse in female.)

4. Venous pattern? (NL no venous bulging.)

5. Obvious pulsations? (NL none.)

b. Arms and legs

1. Size? (NL symmetrical.)

2. Skin color? (NL even distribution of pigment appropriate to genetic heritage and remainder of body. No pallor, cyanosis, or pigment changes.)

3. Hair distribution? (NL present, sparse to dense.)

4. Skin texture? (NL moist, nonfriable appearance.)

5. Venous pattern? (NL no venous bulging.)

6. Obvious pulsations? (NL none.)

7. Edema? (NL none.)

8. Ulcers? (NL none.)

C. *Palpation*

1. *Precordium*: R and L sternal borders, apex, aortic and pulmonic areas.

   a. PMI? (NL 5th LICS MCL—often nonpalpable.)

   b. Lift/heave? (NL none.)

   c. Thrill? (NL none—occasionally felt in normal thin-chested people.) Timing?

2. *Suprasternal notch*: Thrills? (NL none.) Timing?

3. *Neck*, extremities

   a. Arterial pulsations palpated: Carotid (caution: simultaneous bilateral palpation of carotids should not be done), temporal, axillary, brachial, radial, femoral, popliteal, posterior tibial, dorsalis pedis.

   b. Evaluation of pulsations (see fig. 11-2.)

      1. Rate? (NL 60-100 in adults, 70-150 in children varying with age, physical activity, emotional status, muscle

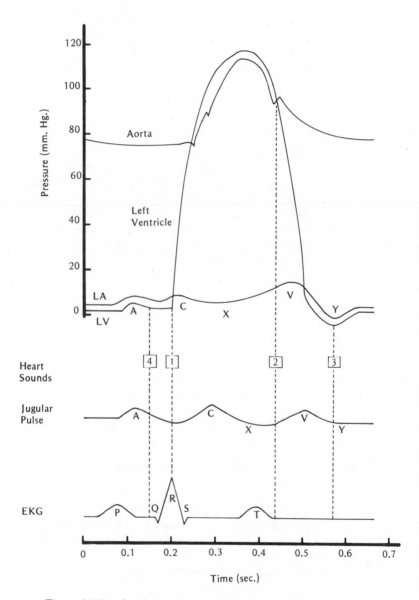

Figure 11-2   Cardiac cycle—arterial and venous pressure curves

tone; no pulse deficit. See normal pulse rates for various
ages, Appendix V.

2. Rhythm? (NL regular. Occasional premature beats not
significant in otherwise healthy client.)

3. Amplitude? (NL all pulses present, symmetrical, amplitude varying with size of artery. No variations in amplitude of single artery beat to beat, pulse character neither
bounding nor thready.
(*Note*: Evaluation scale for recording amplitude: 1+
greatly diminished, 2+ slightly diminished, 3+ normal,
4+ bounding.)

4. Carotid contour? (NL prompt, smooth upstroke not
greater than 0.10 sec duration, descending limb more
gradual.)

c. Elasticity of arterial walls? (NL soft, pliable, not resistent to
compression, not easily rolled between examining fingers,
not tortuous.)

d. Skin temperature? (NL same as rest of body, same both
limbs. Slightly lower skin temperature often reflects superficial vasoconstriction accompanying anxiety, and is of no
significance.)

D. *Percussion*: Cardiac outline—L and R borders of cardiac dullness. (NL
L border cardiac dullness just medial to or at MCL; R border not
normally percussable.)

E. *Auscultation*: Aortic, pulmonic, mitral, tricuspid, left and sternal
border, left axillary, neck and epigastric areas.

1. *Precordium*
a. Heart sounds
1. S_1? (NL "lubb" sound synchronous with carotid
upstroke, louder, duller, lower pitched, and slightly
longer than 2nd sound at apex. Splitting heard normally
in tricuspid area.)

2. S_2? (NL "dupp" sound synchronous with descent of
carotid pulse wave. Louder than first sound at base.

Physiologic splitting of sound normal—heard best at pulmonic area on inspiration. Abnormal if fixed or paradoxical.)

3. S_3? (NL in those otherwise healthy and under 40 years of age. Heard as faint inconstant sound in early diastole with client in L lateral position—louder on expiration and at apex.)

4. S_4? (Generally an abnormal finding. Low-pitched sound heard best at apex. Occurs in late diastole.)

b. Extra sounds

1. Gallops? (NL none.) Accentuated S_3 and S_4 result in gallop rhythms.

   a. Protodiastolic—S_3 (Ken-tuck-y, S_1-S_2-S_3) may be physiologic as found in conditioned athletes, but may represent pathological accentuation as in failing ventricle.

   b. Presystolic—S_4 (Ten-nes-see, S_4-S_1-S_2) almost always pathological.

2. Clicks? (NL none.) Timing?

3. Friction rub? (NL none.) Position? Timing?

c. Murmurs: Diastolic murmurs generally abnormal. Functional murmurs of no significance, sometimes heard in children and young adults as soft, short, early systolic vibratory sounds at pulmonic area or low on LSB which vary with position and respiration. (*Note:* Evaluation scale for recording murmurs: grade 1/6, softest audible; grade 2/6, medium intensity, short duration; grade 3/6, loud, no thrill, moderate duration; grade 4/6, loud, with a thrill, long duration; grade 5/6, loudest heard with stethoscope in chest; grade 6/6, audible with stethoscope off chest.)

1. Site? Radiation?

2. Timing?

3. Pitch?

4. Intensity?

5. Duration?

6. Relationship—position, exercise, respiratory cycle?

7. Character—harsh, blowing, rumbling, crescendo, decrescendo?

   2. *Neck*
      a. Carotid: Bruits? Murmurs? (NL none.)
      b. Jugular: Venous hum? (Generally of no significance. Associated with the functional murmur of childhood.)
   3. *Extremities*: Femoral bruits? (NL none.)

F. **Blood pressure**: Both arms lying, sitting and standing. (NL varies with age; see blood pressure charts, Appendices III and IV. Normal range 100/60 to 140/90 mm Hg, and less than 10 mm Hg difference between limbs. Orthostatic drop should not exceed 10 mm Hg or persist beyond 3 minutes. Thigh blood pressure normally up to 10 mm Hg higher than arm pressure.)

III. LIFE-CYCLE VARIATIONS IN PHYSICAL FINDINGS

A. **Developmental**: Cardiac apex higher in chest in early life. Apical beat in newborn palpated 4th LICS, just lateral to MCL. At age 2 apex reaches 5th LICS. Thick layer of subcutaneous fat makes percussion of little value in assessing infant. Palpation of apical impulse increasingly difficult in adolescents as muscle mass increases in males and breast mass increases in females. Pulse rate drops as cardiac output increases with heart growth. Rate adaption is brisk.

B. **Degenerative**: Heart size decreases with age in the absence of disease. Commonly masking this change is hypertrophy from long-standing hypertension. Shrinkage of vertebral column and neck leads to relative lengthening of aorta, elevations of aortic arch, with rise of innominate artery into the neck. Pulsations therefore are sometimes felt behind clavicular portion of R sternocleidomastoid. In the absence of cardiac hypertrophy, apical impulse may reach LAAL, due to narrowing of rib cage, especially in women. Cardiac output and stroke volume reduced 35% by age 65, but rate at rest unchanged or slightly decreased. With rate adaption diminished and maximal rate reduced, increased time is required to return to resting rate. Blood vessels lose compliance, and peripheral resistance increases, which leads to increased blood pressure and loss in peripheral pulse amplitude. Blood vessels show increasing tortuosity and resistance to compression.

IV. ABNORMAL CONDITIONS

A. Pediatric: Coarctation of aorta, congenital valve stenosis, patent
ductus arteriosis, rheumatic heart disease, septal defects, tetrology of
Fallot.

B. Adult: Angina pectoris, arrhythmias, arterial occlusive disease,
arteriosclerotic heart disease, conduction disturbances, congestive
heart failure, hypertension, valvular disease.

12

Abdomen and Gastrointestinal System

I. HISTORY QUESTIONS

A Change in appetite (Loss = anorexia)? Weight change? Over what time period? How much? Usual diet?

B Difficulty swallowing (dysphagia)? Pain on swallowing?

C Difficulty tolerating any foods?

D Vomiting (emesis)? Nausea? How often? Amount? Color? Odor? Bloody (hematemesis)?

E Indigestion? Use of antacids? How often (frequency)?

F Heartburn (pyrosis)? Belching (eructation)?

G Swollen stomach or bloating after eating (abdominal distention)?

H Burning in pit of stomach (epigastric pain, dyspepsia)?

I Belly pain (abdominal pain)? Where? When? How long? When started? Affected by food? Associated with belching, nerves, stress, fatigue, period (menses)? Intermittent or constant? Cramping (colic)?

J Yellow skin (jaundice)?

K Operations on belly (abdominal surgery)? Names and dates of surgeries? Any problems following surgery?

L Lumps in belly (abdominal masses)?

II CLINICAL EXAMINATION

A. *Preparation*

1. *Position*: Client supine, head on small pillow, arms at sides or across chest, knees may be flexed, breasts and genitals draped.

2. *Equipment*: Stethoscope and tongue blade. Watch, with second hand.

B. Inspection

1. *Skin texture and color?* (NL same as rest of body, not tight or shiny, no discolorations.)

2. *Hair pattern?* (NL sparse to dense in male, soft, light, sparse in female.)

3. *Venous flow pattern?* (NL umbilicus outward.)

4. *Scars, striae, lesions, spider angiomas?* (NL none.)

5. *Contour*, flat, protuberant, gravid, scaphoid? Regional prominences? Adipose distribution? (NL flat, no masses, symmetrical.) Distended? (NL none. Six F's of distension: fat, flatus, feces, fetus, fluid, fibroids.)

6. *Umbilical lesions, herniations? Discolorations?* (NL none.)

7. *Pulsations?* Aorta? Location? (NL epigastrum.)

8. *Fluid wave?* (NL none.)

C. Auscultation: Precedes palpation and percussion in conventional abdominal examination.)

1. *Peristaltic sounds?*
    a. (NL gurgling heard at least every 3-5 seconds, 0.5-second duration.)
    b. (Abnormal: unusually high pitched, rushing, loud, tinkling, especially if associated with pain; absent sounds.)

2. *Bruits?* (NL none.) Aortic? Femoral?

3. *Venous Hum?* (NL none.)

4. *Friction rub?* (NL none.)

5. *Succussion splash?* (NL none.)

D. Percussion: Precedes palpation in conventional abdominal examination.) (See fig 12-1.)

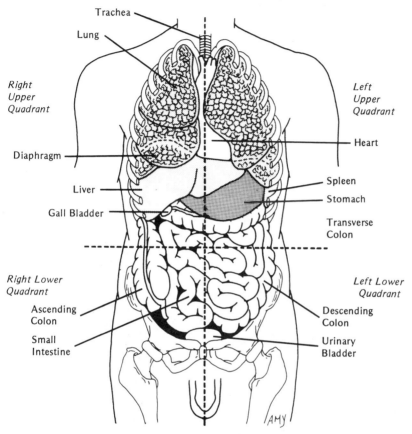

Figure 12-1 Topographical anatomy of the abdomen—anterior

1. *Organ borders?*

   a. Liver dullness: (NL 4–8 cm in midsternal line, 12–15 cm in right midclavicular line.)

   b. Splenic dullness: (NL below 9th interspace posterior to mid-axillary line, and posterior to anterior axillary line on deep inspiration.)

   c. Stomach tympany: (NL in epigastrum and left hypo-chondrium.)

1. *Organ borders*? *cont.*
   d.   Bladder dullness: (NL none, if present found midline in
        suprapubic area if bladder distended.)

2. *Gaseous distention*? (NL none.)

3. *Shifting dullness*? (NL none.)

E. **Palpation** (See fig 12-1, 12-2)

   1. *Pulsation*?
      a.   Aorta: Size? (NL 1-2 cm.) Tenderness? (NL none.)
      b.   Femorals: Presence? (NL bilateral.) Amplitude? (NL strong
           and symmetrical.)

   2. *Tenderness*? (NL none.) Superficial? Deep? Rebound? Point of
      maximum tenderness?

   3. *Rigidity*? Guarding? (NL none.)

   4. *Masses*?
      a.   Liver: (Usually nonpalpable. If palpable, liver edge is smooth,
           firm, sharp, nontender, just under the costal margin.)
      b.   Spleen: (NL nonpalpable, nontender.)
      c.   Kidneys: (Usually nonpalpable, if palpable lower pole right
           kidney 4 cm above iliac crest at right midinguinal line, poles
           descend on deep inspiration. NL nontender.)
      d.   Gallbladder: (NL nonpalpable, nontender.)
      e.   Descending colon: (NL firmness from collected fecal
           matter.)
      f.   Other masses: (NL none.) Size? Location? Tenderness? Con-
           sistency? Pulsation? Fixation? Relationship to abdominal
           organs? Move with respiration?

   5. *Superficial skin reflexes*? (NL brief movement of umbilicus
      toward side of stimulation.)

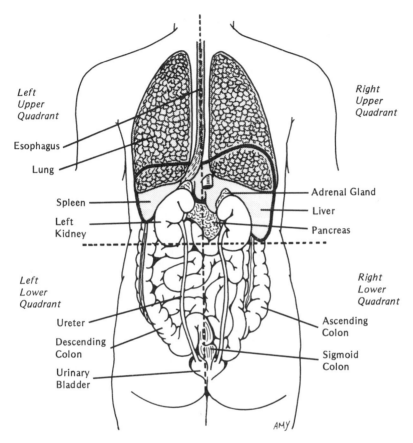

Left
Upper
Quadrant

Right
Upper
Quadrant

Esophagus

Lung

Spleen

Left
Kidney

Adrenal Gland

Liver

Pancreas

Left
Lower
Quadrant

Right
Lower
Quadrant

Ureter

Descending
Colon

Urinary
Bladder

Ascending
Colon

Sigmoid
Colon

AMY

Figure 12-2   Topographical anatomy of the abdomen—posterior

III. LIFE-CYCLE VARIATIONS IN PHYSICAL FINDINGS

*A.   **Developmental***: Umbilical cord remnant in neonates falls off within 2
weeks. Disproportionate abdominal size and pot-bellied appearance in
infancy and toddlerhood gives way to slimming of torso usually by
age 5. Growth of trunk is proportionate to growth of body. Superficial abdominal venous pattern is observable until puberty. Liver is

often palpable in infants and young children and may be felt up to 3 finger breadths below the costal margin. Spleen tip and both kidneys are also often palpable in infants. The bladder in infants may be felt and percussed in the level of the umbilicus.

B. *Degenerative*: Reduced circulation to abdominal organs from arteriosclerotic vascular narrowing. Occlusion manifests in changes in organ function and reduction in size. Loss of diaphragmatic muscle tone leads to formation of hiatal hernias. Loss of skin elasticity leads to skin redundancy.

IV. ABNORMAL CONDITIONS

A. *Pediatric*: Appendicitis, colitis, constipation, gastroenteritis, infectious hepatitis, malabsorption syndromes, splenomegaly due to infectious mononucleosis, umbilical hernias, Wilms's tumor.

B. *Adult*: Appendicitis, atrophic gastritis, constipation, intestinal angina, lymphoma, malabsorption, neoplasms of stomach, large intestines, ovary, and bladder, peptic ulcer, regional enteritis, ulcerative colitis.

13
Anus and Rectum

I. HISTORY QUESTIONS

A Loose bowel movement (diarrhea)? Frequent BM? Bloody or black BM (melena)?

B BM's regular? Constipated? Recent change? BM's hard or soft? Frothy BM's (steatorrhea)?

C Use laxatives or enemas? What kind? How often?

D Pass gas frequently (flatulence)?

E Pain during BM (dyschezia)? Pus or mucus in BM? Feel need to pass BM frequently, without result (tenesmus)?

F Itching of anus (anal pruritis)? Burning? Pain? Spasm?

G Hemorrhoids? Remedy?

H Soiling problem (fecal incontinence)?

II. CLINICAL EXAMINATION

A. *Preparation*

1. *Position*: Adolescents and adults: (1) torso prone across examining table, hips flexed, feet on floor; (2) lateral or Sim's position with hip and knee flexed and buttocks close to the edge of examining table; (3) dorsolithotomy position. Female examination often done with examination of genitalia. Infants and older children: supine with examiner holding feet with one hand in midline position with knees and hips flexed onto abdomen.

2. *Equipment*: Glove or finger cots, lubricant, good lighting.

B. Inspection

1. *Anus and perianal area*
    a. Color? Texture? (NL more pigmented and coarser than surrounding skin.)
    b. Hair pattern, density, texture? (NL sparse circumanal hair, coarse and kinky in appearance.)
    c. Lesions, scars, fissures? (NL none.) Location?
    d. Rashes, excoriation, inflammation? (NL none.)
    e. Lumps, fistulas, hemorrhoids, prolapse? (NL none.)

2. *Rectum*—the Valsalva maneuver
    a. Fissures, hemorrhoids, polyps? (NL none.)
    b. Prolapse? (NL none.)

3. *Pilonidal area*
    a. Dimples, inflammation, sinus opening, discharge? (NL none.)
    b. Hair density? (NL none to moderate.)

C. Palpation

1. *Anal sphincter*
    a. Tone? (NL tightens, then relaxes to allow insertion of finger or probe. No stricture or failure of tightening response.)
    b. Internal hemorrhoids? (NL none.)
    c. Tenderness, nodules? (NL none.)

2. *Rectum*
    a. Male and female examination: Posterior and lateral rectal walls.
        1. Consistency? (NL smooth, with no nodules, polyps, or masses.)
        2. Tenderness? (NL none.)
    b. Male examination
        1. Prostate
            a. Size? (NL 4 cm in diameter.)
            b. Shape? (NL symmetrical, bilobed with median sulcus.)
            c. Consistency? (NL firm, rubbery, and smooth.)

      d.   Location? (NL anterior rectal wall.)

      e.   Mobility? (NL not completely fixed.)

      f.   Tenderness? (NL none if palpated with light pressure.)

      g.   Discharge? (NL none produced through urinary meatus after light massage.)

  2.   Seminal vesicles: (NL frequently nonpalpable.)

      a.   Location? (NL anterior rectal wall, above and lateral to prostate.)

      b.   Consistency? (NL slightly corrugated.)

      c.   Tenderness? (NL none.)

  c. Female examination

    1.   Cervix

      a.   Shape? (NL small, round mass.)

      b.   Location? (NL anterior rectal wall.)

    2.   Uterus: (NL nonpalpable from rectum; if moderately retroflexed, uterus palpable on anterior rectal wall.)

    3.   Pilonidal area: (NL nontender, no induration or swelling.)

D. *Percussion and auscultation*: Not part of the conventional anal and rectal examination.

E. *Fecal examination*

  1. *Color*? (NL dark brown. No absence of color, no tarry or bloody color.)

  2. *Consistency*? (NL soft, maintaining constant shape, no mucus, not watery, stony, frothy.)

  3. *Smear for occult blood.*

III. LIFE-CYCLE VARIATIONS IN PHYSICAL FINDINGS

A. *Developmental*: Bowel control should be achieved by age 3. Digital rectal examinations on infants and children are done only when there is a history of bleeding, pain, or severe, constant constipation. Anal hair may appear at puberty.

B. **Degenerative**: Loss of abdominal muscle tone, relaxation of the pelvic floor, and insufficient intake of bulk-producing foods cause constipation, and sometimes hard rectal masses are palpated in the LLQ. Decreased rectal sensation to balloon distension and loss of anal sphincter tone may be associated with incontinence. Loss of sphincter tone may be apparent on digital examination. The prostate is often enlarged, and in the benign state is palpated as a firm, smooth, symmetrical, slightly elastic enlargement. It may bulge more than a centimeter into the rectal lumen and obliterate the median sulcus, but should not obstruct urinary flow.

IV. ABNORMAL CONDITIONS

A. **Pediatric**: Anal fissure, imperforate anus, pilonidal sinus and cyst, prolapsed rectum, rashes.

B. **Adult**: Anorectal fistula, benign and malignant prostatic hypertrophy, carcinoma, fissures, internal and external hemorrhoids, incompetent sphincter, ischiorectal abscess, pilonidal cyst, polyps, prolapse of rectum, pruritis ani, prostatitis, stricture of rectum.

14

Female Genitalia and Reproductive System

I. HISTORY QUESTIONS

A   Difficulty passing water (voiding, urination, micturition)? Painful (dysuria)? Burning sensation? Unable to wait to urinate even when bladder not full (urgency)? Passing water in small amounts often (frequency)? Blood in urine (hematuria)? Urine color?

B   How often pass water? Amount? Awaken during night to pass water (nocturia)? How many times?

C   Difficulty starting a stream? Difficulty stopping a stream? Change in force of stream? Any dribbling?

D   Problem wetting self (incontinence)? Pass water on laughing, sneezing, coughing, or bearing down (stress incontinence)? Pass water while sleeping (enuresis)?

E   Problem with kidney stones (renal calculi)? Gravel in urine?

F   Bladder infection after intercourse? How often?

G   Discharge from vagina? Color? Consistency? Odor? Amount?

H   Contact with syphilis, gonorrhea, or other venereal disease?

I   Sores on vagina?

J   Age at first period (menarche)? Length of cycle? Duration of flow? Interval between periods? Pain or cramps (dysmenorrhea)? Remedies tried? Regular (catamenia)? Date last period began (LMP)? Excessive flow (menorrhagia)? Bleeding between periods (metrorrhagia)?

K   Ever pregnant? How many times? Any complications? Type delivery? Number of living children? Abortions or miscarriages?
    (Note: Record as (Gr) (Gravida number?)_____(Para number?)
    _____ (Full term number?); _____(Premature number?); _____
    (Abortion number?); _____(Living children number?)

L   Date last Pap smear? Result?

M   Vaginal or uterine surgery?

N   Date period stopped (menopause)? Any bleeding since then?

O   Problems with intercourse? Painful (dyspareunia)? Frequency of intercourse (libido)? Bleeding after intercourse (postcoital bleeding)?

P   Type of contraception?

Q   Problem getting pregnant (infertility)?

II. CLINICAL EXAMINATION

A. *Preparation*

1. *Position*: Dorsolithotomy

2. *Client preparation*: Client directed not to douche for 24 hours prior to examination and to empty bladder just before examination. Undergarments removed and draped from waist down.

3. *Equipment*: Gloves, adjustable light, vaginal speculum of appropriate size, sterile cotton topped applicators, spatula, glass slides, fixation solution, and lubrication jelly.

B. *Inspection*

1. *Structures visualized*: mons pubis, clitoris, labia majora, labia minora, vestibule, urethral meatus, introitus, fourchette, perineal body. (See fig 14-1.)

2. *External observations*
    a. Hair pattern? (NL dense, coarse, kinky hair growing in inverted triangular pattern. Sparse hair on upper thighs normal.)
    b. Lesions? Edema? Erythema? Inflammation? Lacerations? Smegma? Cysts? Masses? Vesicles? Chancres? Increased Pigmentation? Discharge? (NL none.) Color? Amount? Odor? Consistency?
    c. Scars? (Perineal scars frequently seen in primiparous and multiparous women.)
    d. Incontinence on bearing down? (NL none.)

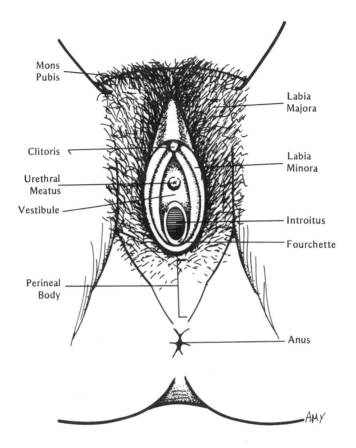

Figure 14-1   External female genitalia

e.   Prolapse of vaginal wall? (NL none.)

3.   *Internal observations*: The speculum examination (See fig. 14-2.)
    a.   Cervix
        1.   Color? (NL pink.)
        2.   Diameter (NL 2–3 cm.)
        3.   Erosion? Ulcer? Masses? Cysts? Inflammation? Old lacerations? (NL none.)

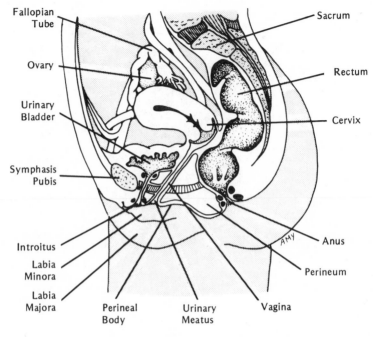

Figure 14-2   Cross section female genitalia

  4. Discharge? (NL small amount clear mucus.)
 b. Cervical os
  1. Size? (NL 3 to 5 mm in diameter, note stenosis.)
  2. Shape? (NL round dimple-nulliparous cervix, slit-parous cervix. See fig. 14-3.)
  3. Polyps? (NL none.)
  4. Erosion? (NL none to small amount.)
  5. Bleeding? (NL none.)
  6. Eversion? (NL none.)
 c. Vagina
  1. Color? (NL pink, bluish cast normal prior to menses, and in pregnancy.)
  2. Texture? (NL smooth folds.)
  3. Bulging, cysts, masses, ulcerations? (NL none.)
  4. Discharge? (NL clear mucus.) Color? Amount? Odor?

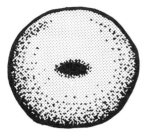
Nulliparous Cervix

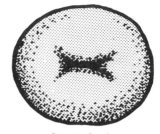
Parous Cervix

Figure 14-3   Nulliparous and parous cervix

C. *Palpation*:   Bimanual examination

1. *Cervix*
    a. Position? (NL posterior from top to anterior vaginal wall.)
    b. Consistency? (NL similar to tip of nose with a dimple.)
    c. Mobility? (NL freely movable for 2 to 3 cm in any direction.)
    d. Tenderness, nodules? (NL none.)

2. *Uterus*
    a. Size? (NL 5 cm long, 4 cm wide, and 2.5 cm thick.)
    b. Position? (NL anteflexed in midline, retroflexion normal if position not fixed.)
    c. Contour? (NL smooth, inverted pear.)
    d. Consistency? (NL firm.)
    e. Mobility? (NL freely movable.)
    f. Tenderness? (NL none.)

3. *Uterine adnexa*
    a. Fallopian tubes? (NL not palpable.)
    b. Ovary
        1. Size? (NL 3.5 to 4 cm long, 2 cm wide, and 1.5 cm thick.)
        2. Contour? (NL smooth, almond shaped.)
        3. Mobility? (NL very mobile.)
        4. Tenderness? (NL some.)

4. *Cul de sac area*
   a. Masses? (NL none.)
   b. Bulging? (NL none.)
   c. Tenderness? (NL none.)

D. *Percussion and auscultation*: Not part of the conventional genitalia examination.

E. *Papanicolaou smear*: Vaginal, cervical, and endocervical smears.

III. LIFE-CYCLE VARIATIONS IN PHYSICAL FINDINGS

A. *Developmental*: Newborn labia minora are prominent and a bloody vaginal discharge may be apparent for the 1st week of life, changing to serosanguinous for another 1–2 weeks. Growth of genitalia in childhood is proportionate to body size. Pubic hair appears in pubescent females ages 8–13 in a characteristic triangular pattern, and the onset of menses occurs between ages 9 and 17, with an increase in vaginal secretions. Diurnal bladder control by age 3 and nocturnal bladder control by age 4½.

B. *Pregnancy*: Prominent softened, dusky blue cervix; cyanosis of upper vaginal tissue; enlarged, softer uterus; enlarged, firmer lower abdomen. Increased clear vaginal discharge, cervical os elliptical.

C. *Degenerative*: Sparse, gray vulvar hair; labial shrinking, thin atrophic vaginal wall; smooth, dry, red vaginal mucosa along with shortening and narrowing of the vaginal canal. Decreased perineal tone occurs as well as scarring of posterior fourchette from episeotomy.

IV. ABNORMAL CONDITIONS

A. *Pediatric*: Ambiguous genitalia, foreign bodies in vagina, labial adhesions, precocious puberty.

B. *Adult*: Candida albicans, cervical polyps, cervicitis, cystocele, gonorrhea, inflammation of Bartholin's gland, ovarian cyst, prolapsed uterus, rectocele, retrodisplacement of uterus, syphilis, trichomonas vaginalis, tumors, uterine fibroids, urethral caruncle.

15
Male Genitalia

I. HISTORY QUESTIONS

A Difficulty passing water (voiding, urination, micturition)? Painful (dysuria)? Burning sensation? Unable to wait to void (urgency)? Blood in urine (hematuria)? Urine color?

B How often pass water each day (frequency)? Amount? Awaken during night to pass water (nocturia)? How many times?

C Problem wetting self (incontinence)? Problem getting to the bathroom on time (urgency incontinence)? Pass water on laughing, sneezing, coughing, or bearing down (stress incontinence)? Pass water during sleep (enuresis)?

D Difficulty starting a stream? Difficulty stopping a stream? Change in force of stream? Weak stream? Dribbling? Feeling of incomplete emptying of bladder?

E Problems with kidney stones (renal calculi)? Gravel in urine? Back pain (flank pain)?

F Prostate trouble?

G Rashes, sores, ulcers, blisters on penis or scrotum? Painful?

H Discharge? Color? Amount? Odor?

I Contact with venereal disease?

J Painful testes? Swelling? Lumps?

K Change in sex drive (libido)? Able to achieve erection? Able to achieve ejaculation?

II. CLINICAL EXAMINATION

A. *Preparation*

1. *Position*: Client in supine and standing positions.
2. *Equipment*: Stool for examiner. Gloves for examiner where danger of cross-infection.

B. *Inspection*

1. *Pubic hair*: (NL present, often in diamond shaped distribution, with dense coarse curly hairs extending up to umbilicus and down to upper thighs. Absence or extreme sparseness of pubic hair abnormal. Presence of hair on penile shaft abnormal.)

2. *Penis*
   a. Size? (NL proportionate to body size, no virilism, no infantilism.)
   b. Foreskin retraction? (NL foreskin, if present, retracts with ease. No phimosis, paraphimosis, or smegma.)
   c. Location of urinary meatus? (NL central position at tip of glans penis. No displacement proximally along shaft or to superior or inferior surfaces of shaft. See fig. 15-1.)
   d. Inflammation, edema, and/or erythema? (NL none on glans or penile shaft.)
   e. Scars, rashes, excoriations, nodules, warts, other painful or nontender lesions? (NL none on glans or penile shaft.)
   f. Discharge? (NL none.) Color? Amount? Odor?

3. *Scrotum* (See fig. 15-2)
   a. Shape? (NL pear shaped, usually asymmetrical with left testis lower than right.)
   b. Skin appearance? (NL sometimes slightly darker in pigment, lying in loose transverse folds.)
   c. Hair distribution? (NL present but scant.)
   d. Venous pattern? (NL nonengorged, no varicose veins.)
   e. Scars, rashes, nodules, lumps, ulcers, excoriations? (NL none.)
   f. Inflammation, edema, and/or erythema? (NL none.)

g. Discharge? (NL none.) Color? Amount? Odor?

h. Transillumination? (NL not translucent if testes present and not enlarged.)

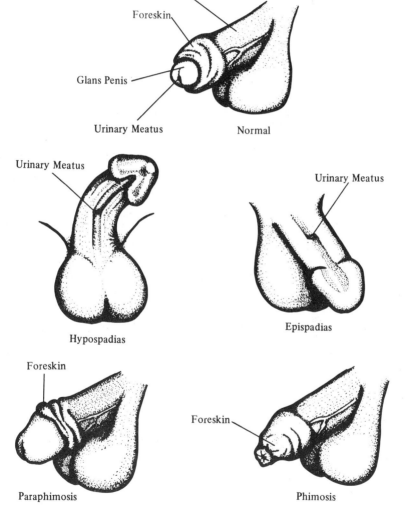

Figure 15-1 Abnormalities of urethral meatus and foreskin

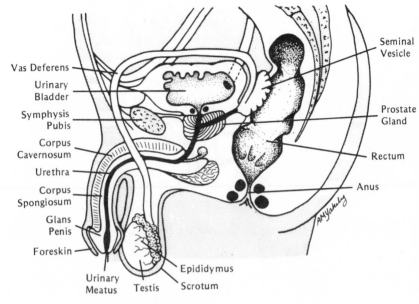

Figure 15-2   Cross section male pelvic organs

C. Palpation

1. *Penis*
   a. Masses? (NL none on glans or penile shaft.)
   b. Tenderness, and/or induration? (NL none on glans or penile shaft.)
   c. Expressible urethral secretion? (NL none.)

2. *Scrotum* (See fig. 15-2.)
   a. Testes
      1. Presence? (NL palpable.)
      2. Size? (NL 4 by 3 by 2.5 cm, small variation not abnormal.)
      3. Shape? (NL ovoid.)
      4. Consistency? (NL firm, smooth, rubbery.)

   5. Mobility? (NL freely movable in scrotal sac.)

   6. Tenderness? (NL tender with application of moderate pressure.)

  b. Epididymis

   1. Shape? (NL crescent.)

   2. Position? (NL on posterior aspect of testes.)

   3. Scarring, swelling, masses? (NL none.)

   4. Tenderness? (NL none.)

  c. Spermatic cord

   1. Masses? (NL none.)

   2. Tender? (NL nontender.)

 3. *Inguinal canal*

  a. Inguinal hernia? (NL none.) Direct? Indirect?

  b. Dilitation of inguinal ring? (NL none.)

  c. Weakness of inguinal ring? (NL none.)

 4. *Femoral canal*? (NL no herniation.)

D. ***Percussion and auscultation***: Not part of conventional genitalia examination.

E. ***Cremasteric reflex***: (NL prompt elevation of testes on side of stimulus.)

III. LIFE-CYCLE VARIATIONS IN PHYSICAL FINDINGS

A. ***Developmental:*** The cremasteric reflex is very brisk in infant and young males, and may give false impression of undescended testes. Growth of penis and scrotal sac is proportionate to body size prior to puberty, then disproportionate in early puberty, giving the appearance of larger genitals. Pubic hair appears at approximately age 10. Diurnal bladder control achieved by age 3, and nocturnal control by age 4½.

B. ***Degenerative***: Graying and thinning of pubic hair occurs in 5th and 6th decades. Slight testicular atrophy may be present in 7th and 8th decades.

IV. ABNORMAL CONDITIONS

A. ***Pediatric***: Epispadius, hydrocele, hypospadius, infantilism, inguinal hernia, torsion of appendix testis, torsion of spermatic cord, undescended testicle, virilism chordee.

B. ***Adult***: Balanoposthitis, condyloma acuminatum, epididymitis, hydrocele, incontinence, inguinal hernia, neoplasm, orchitis, paraphimosis, phimosis, Peyronie's disease, scrotal cyst, spermatocele, syphilis, torsion of spermatic cord, torsion of testes, varicocele.

16
Musculoskeletal System

I. HISTORY QUESTIONS

A   Stiffness, pain, weakness in joints or muscles? Which joints or muscles involved? Related to activity? Occur at rest? Time of day?

B   Swollen joints? Red or hot joints?

C   Ever told have rheumatism or gout?

D   Difficulty getting out of bed? Off chair? Combing hair? Brushing teeth? Feeding self? (Problems with ADL.)

E   Difficulty walking? Reason? Movement limited? How? Pain in hip or grating sensation when walking? Grating sensation when moving any joint? Limp?

F   Pain, stiffness, or cramping in calves? Occur with walking or other physical exercise (intermittent claudication)? Occur suddenly? One leg or both? Night pain?

G   Broken bones (fractures)? Joint dislocation? Sprains or strains? How many? Where? Bone deviations—bowlegs, knock-knees?

H   Back pain? Associated with numbness or tingling of leg? When does it come on (onset)? Travel down your leg (radiate)? Increase with coughing, laughing, or bearing down (radicular pain)?

I   Any muscles look smaller (atrophy)? Do you consider yourself handicapped?

J   Feet painful? Trouble with corns or bunions?

II. CLINICAL EXAMINATION

A. *Preparation*

1. *Position*: Client in upright position, loosely draped.
2. *Equipment*: Adequate room lighting, cloth tape measure, goniometer if available.

B. *Inspection*

1. *Total body*? (NL no gross asymmetry of one side as compared to other, no gross deformities, skin lesions, swellings or masses. Slight asymmetries of no pathological significance.)

2. *Thorax and back*
    a. Posture? (NL erect, head balanced midway between level shoulders, shoulders aligned plumb with hips, hips centered over knees and ankles. Pelvis level in erect and flexed position.)
    b. Contour of back? (NL cervical curve concave, thoracic curve convex, lumbar curve concave, with a straight midspinal line. No lateral curvature (scoliosis), exaggeration of thoracic convexity (kyphosis), lumbar concavity (lordosis), or humpback (gibbus).
    c. Range of motion
        1. Mobility of dorsal spine? (NL with ease and no pain able to elevate and depress shoulders, rotate shoulders forward and back 30 degrees, rotate shoulders in arc 360 degrees.)
        2. Mobility of lumbar spine? (NL with ease and no pain able to bend forward at waist 75–90 degrees, and backward 30 degrees; able to twist at waist 30 degrees forward and back; able to bend laterally 35 degrees.)
        3. Straight leg raising test? (NL no pain on flexation of hips to 90 degrees.)
    d. Position of scapulae? (NL symmetrical, no elevation or winging.)
    e. Chest expansion? (NL nipple line 3 cm larger on full inspiration.)

3. *Extremities*
    a. Length and diameter? (NL consistent with genetic heritage, symmetrical to 1 mm difference, arm span equal to height.)
    b. Extremity mass? (NL proportionate to body size. No acromegaly, edema, or local masses.)
    c. Muscle condition? (NL dominant limb may have slightly greater muscular development. No contractures, hypertrophy in the absence of conditioning, atrophy or fasciculations.)
    d. Bone and joint formation? (NL symmetrical, no swelling, discoloration, masses, nodules. No deviation away from midline—valgus, or toward midline—varus.)
    e. Range of motion? (NL considerable variation of joint tightness. Joint hyperextension not necessarily pathologically significant.)
        1. Arm
            a. Mobility of shoulders? (NL able to shrug shoulders—Cranial Nerve XI, Accessory.)
                1. Adduction? (NL 50 degrees.)
                2. Abduction? (NL 180 degrees.)
                3. External rotation? (NL 90 degrees.)
                4. Internal rotation? (NL 90 degrees.)
                5. Forward flexion? (NL 180 degrees.)
                6. Extension? (NL 50 degrees.)
            b. Elbow
                1. Flexion? (NL 160 degrees.)
                2. Extension? (NL 0 degrees.)
                3. Supination? (NL palm up, 90 degrees.)
                4. Pronation? (NL palm down, 90 degrees.)
             c. Wrist
                1. Radial deviation? (NL 20 degrees.)
                2. Ulnar deviation? (NL 55 degrees.)
                3. Flexion? (NL 90 degrees.)
                4. Extension? (NL 70 degrees.)
             d. Fingers
                1. Metacarpophalangeal
                    a. Flexion? (NL fingertip touch distal palmar crease, 90 degrees.)
                    b. Hyperextension? (NL 30 degrees.)

        2. Proximal interphalangeal
           a. Flexion? (NL 120 degrees.)
           b. Extension? (NL 0 degrees.)
        3. Distal interphalangeal
           a. Flexion? (NL 80 degrees.)
           b. Extension? (NL 0 degrees.)

2. Hip
    a. Knee straight
        1. Flexion? (NL 90 degrees.)
        2. Hyperextension? (NL 15 degrees.)
    b. Knee bent
        1. Flexion? (NL 120 degrees.)
        2. Extension? (NL 0 degrees.)
    c. Abduction? (NL 45 degrees.)
    d. Adduction? (NL 30 degrees.)
    e. Internal rotation? (NL 20–40 degrees.)
    f. External rotation? (NL 45 degrees.)

3. Leg
    a. Knee
        1. Hyperextension? (NL 15 degrees.)
        2. Flexion? (NL 130 degrees.)
    b. Ankles
        1. Dorsiflexion? (NL 20 degrees, toward head.)
        2. Plantar flexion? (NL 45 degrees, away from head.)
        3. Inversion? (NL 30 degrees.)
        4. Eversion? (NL 20 degrees.)

4. *Movement–general*
    a. Type of gait? (NL fluid, balanced, coordinated walking movements. No unusually short steps, wide based walk, restricted swinging of arms, staggering, trunkal lurching, dragging of feet, or watching feet while walking. No toeing in, toeing out, drop foot, antalgic, trendelenberg, spastic, or scissor gait.)
    b. General? (NL with smooth coordinated movement, no pain, and only minimal assistance, able to get on and off examining table, onto and up from chair, roll from side to side, sit up from lying position.)

C. Palpation

1. *Muscles*
    a. Tone? (NL slight resistance to passive movement despite voluntary relaxation; no spasticity, no rigidity, no excessive firmness or flabbiness.)
    b. Fasciculations? (NL none.)
    c. Masses? (NL none.)
    d. Tenderness? (NL none.)

2. *Joints*
    a. Temperature? (NL same as rest of body.)
    b. Crepitation? (NL none.)
    c. Masses, swelling, capsular thickening? (NL none.)
    d. Tenderness? (NL none.)

3. *Bone*: (NL firm, no tenderness or masses, no abnormal prominences.)

D. Percussion

1. *Spine*? (NL nontender.)

2. *Costovertebral angle*? (NL nontender.)

E. Auscultation: Not part of conventional musculoskeletal examination.

F. Assessment of Muscle Strength: (NL no weakness, if present, note if proximal or distal.)

1. *Fingers*? (NL able to straighten and flex against resistance.)

2. *Biceps and Triceps*? (NL able to maintain partially extended position of the arm against pushing and pulling forces.)

3. *Shoulders*? (NL able to shrug shoulders against resistance.)

4. *Abdominal*? (NL able to raise from supine to sitting without support.)

5. *Back extensions*? (NL able to raise head and shoulders while lying prone.)

6. *Thigh and hip*? (NL able to flex against resistance.)

7. *Thigh adductors*: (NL able to maintain tight knees against pulling.)

8. *Thigh abductors*? (NL able to maintain knee abduction against pushing.)

9. *Quadraceps*? (NL able to extend knees against resistance, able to rise from deep knee bend.)

10. *Feet*? (NL able to plantar and dorsiflex against resistance, able to toe and heel walk.)

III. LIFE-CYCLE VARIATIONS IN PHYSICAL FINDINGS

A. *Developmental*

1. *Infancy*: Bones very soft and flexible, composed mainly of cartilage, and joints are elastic. Back straight and flat; lumbar and sacral curves develop from age 6–12 months. Legs short, small, and bowed; feet flat, and toeing in and toeing out are frequent. In the absence of significant pathology, ages 1 through adolescence may show increased internal rotation of hips (up to 60 degrees) which gradually decreases with age. Arms and fingers are short. Muscles of extremities resist passive movement. Movements are random and uncoordinated. Muscular development proceeds cephalocaudally and from the center to the periphery. See emerging patterns of behavior during the 1st year of life, see Appendix VII. Rate of growth rapid.

2. *Toddlerhood to late childhood*: Slower rate of physical growth and motor development. Increased strength, skill and coordination. See emerging patterns of development from 1 to 5 years of age, see Appendix VIII.

3. *Puberty*: Rapid physical growth resumes with bones growing faster than muscles which often leads to clumsiness and poor posture. Large muscles grow faster than smaller ones which causes lack of coordination. Extremities and hands and feet may grow out of proportion to remainder of body. In females there is an increase in the absolute and relative width of the pelvis. In males there is an expansion of muscle mass, particularly in later adolescence, along with an increase in absolute and relative shoulder breadth from age 13 on.

B. *Pregnancy*: In the third trimester there is an exaggeration of the lumbar curve and a temporary lordosis results.

C. *Degenerative*: Atrophy of bone may cause loss of height, particularly in women. Decreased physical strength may be apparent in muscle strength resistance tests. Calcification of the articular cartilage can occur, as well as of the menisci of the knee joints. This causes a loss of cartilage resilience, but usually no change in range of motion, though ease of movement may be diminished. Loss in range of motion occurs with aging. Characteristically it should not have a rapid onset, be associated with pain, or interfere with ADL. Often there is thoracic kyphosis with decrease in height, and arm span increases relative to height. Slight standing hip and knee flexion is often apparent in the 7th decade.

IV. ABNORMAL CONDITIONS

A. *Pediatric*: Club foot, Colles fracture, congenital hip dislocation, cubitus valgus, cubitus varus, genu valgus, genu varus, kyphosis, Legg-Perthes disease, macrodactyly, scoliosis, slipped epiphysis, super-numery digits, torticollis, webbed digits, webbing of toes.

B. *Adult*: Arthritis, bunion, bursitis, carpel tunnel syndrome, Charot's joint, corns, floating patella, frozen shoulder, ganglion, hallux valgus, hammer toe, hip fracture, knee cartilage and ligament trauma, meniscus and ligament trauma, nucleus pulposus, pes cavus, pes planus, spontaneous rupture of biceps, supraspinatus tendon syndrome, tendonitis, tennis synovitis, wrist drop.

17
Neurologic System and Psychiatric Examination

I. HISTORY QUESTIONS

A. *Neurologic*

A Headaches? How often? Where? Occurs with what—nausea, vomiting, sinus tenderness, emotional upset?

B Dizziness or vertigo?

C Ever feel faint (syncope)? Blackout? When? How often? Occurs with what?

D Fits or convulsions (seizure, epilepsy)? Started when? How often? Accompanied by any special feeling (aura)? On medication?

E Sudden jerks (twitching)? Where? Noticed when?

F More difficulty than usual remembering? Noticed when?

G Problem swallowing (dysphagia)? Noticed when?

H Problem speaking or talking (dysphasia, dysarthria)? Trouble reading? Noticed when?

I Handwriting changes (dysgraphia)? Noticed when?

J Any body part numb (anesthesia)? Tingle or feel like pins and needles (paresthesia)?

K Problem moving any part of body (paresis, paralysis)?

L Problem with coordination (dysmetria, dyssynergia)?

M Tendency to shake or tremble (tremors)? Noticed when?

N Change in ability to control bowel or bladder (incontinence)?

O Change in vision? Blind spots (scotoma)? Where (location in visual field)? Occur with what?

P History of significant head or nerve injury? When? After effects (sequelae)?

B. *Psychiatric*

A   Any emotional problems? Often anxious? Tense?
B   Tend to worry a lot?
C   Problems falling asleep or staying asleep (insomnia)?
D   Difficulty relaxing (anxiety)?
E   Annoyed by little things?
F   Dislike criticism?
G   Lose temper often?
H   Disturbed by work, family, or health problems?
I   Sexual difficulties?
J   Ever sought psychological counseling or psychiatric help?
K   Ever considered or attempted suicide or homicide? How?
L   Tend to be shy or sensitive?
M   Nervous around strangers?
N   Anything in your surroundings have special meaning for you it does not have for other people (ideas of reference)?
O   Do you feel you have special powers or beliefs others do not have (delusions)?
P   Ever hear voices when no one is there? Ever see things that are not there (hallucinations)?
Q   Ever feel that you are being plotted against or persecuted (paranoia)?

II. CLINICAL EXAMINATION

A. *Preparation*

1. *Position*: Client should be physically and psychologically comfortable.

2. *Equipment*: Reflex hammer, tuning fork, safety pin, cotton ball, eye chart, ophthalmoscope, watch and Denver Developmental Screening Test kit or equivalent for testing children.

B. *Mental Status Assessment*

1. *Level of consciousness*? (NL fully alert on arousal, normal sleep-awake pattern, no lethargy, no fluctuation in LOC.)

2. *Orientation*? (NL unhesitatingly state person, place, date, situation.)

3. *Mood and behavior*? (NL attentive to examiner, not hostile, agitated, hypoactive, bizarre. No delusions, illusions, hallucinations. Pattern appropriate to age, status, background and sex.)

4. *Knowledge and vocabulary*? (NL appropriate to age, education, cultural background, life experiences. Able to name five objects in familiar category and recognize five familiar symbols.)

5. *Judgment and abstraction*? (NL able to form appropriate genera ization when presented with several specific items in a category. Able to discern abstract meaning of simple proverb. Able to plot sensible course of action.)

6. *Memory*
   a. Immediate recall? (NL can repeat seven digits forward and four backward.)
   b. Recent memory? (NL after 5-minute time lapse can remember 3 objects presented.)
   c. Remote memory? (NL recall of past events intact.)

7. *Calculation?* (NL able to perform simple math exercises, able to subtract serial 7s.)

C. *Language and speech*

1. *Speech*? (NL clearly articulated, no slurring, no bizarre intonations.)

2. *Language*? (NL able to use and interpret language with ease, no difficulty sending or receiving verbal, written, or gestural messages.)

D. *Special cortical functions*? (NL no visual, auditory, or tactile agnosias, no body image difficulties.)

E. *Cranial nerves*? Testing done conventionally as part of HEENT examination. (See cranial nerve chart, table 17-1, for summary of cranial nerve function.)

F. *Cerebellar assessment*

1. *Balance*
    a. Gait? (NL coordinated, smooth, not Parkinsonian, ataxic: no wide stance, trunkal lurching, staggering, limping, or unequal arm swing.)
    b. Romberg? (NL no wavering of station or posture with eyes closed, arms outstretched, feet together.)
2. *Coordination*
    a. Finger-to-nose? (NL no past pointing.)
    b. Heel-to-shin? (NL smooth accurate movements.)
    c. Alternating motion? (NL smooth, coordinated, rapid forearm supination and pronation.)
    d. Tandem walking? (NL able to take several steps without lurching, reeling, or widening stance.)

G. *Motor assessment*

1. *Muscles*
    a. Size? (NL full development. No wasting or flabby hypertrophy.)
    b. Symmetry? (NL symmetrical.)
    c. Tone? (NL slight resistance to passive movement despite voluntary relaxation. No spasticity or rigidity, excessive firmness or flabbiness.)
    d. Strength? (NL able to resist opposing force appropriately with all muscle groups.)

2. *Movement* (NL voluntary control intact, no tics, muscle fibrillation and fasciculation, tremors, twitches, or convulsions.)
    a. Start where? Local or general?
    b. Continuous or intermittent?
    c. Occur at rest?
    d. Accompany voluntary movement?
    e. Fine? Coarse?

TABLE 17-1: Cranial Nerves

Nerve	Function	Normal Response
Cranial I: Olfactory	Smell.	Eyes closed, correctly differentiates familiar odors with each nostril.
Cranial II: Optic	Visual acuity.	Accurately calls out letters on 20/20 test line of eye chart.
	Color vision.	Differentiates between red and green lines on Snellen chart.
	Near vision.	Able to read newsprint at distance of 1 ft. or 30 cm.
	Peripheral vision.	Identifies object 60 degrees nasalward, 50 degrees upward, 90 degrees temporally, 70 degrees downward.
Cranial III: Oculomotor	Pupillary reactivity.	Pupil size symmetrical, neither widely dilated nor pinpoint in average room light. Prompt constriction in reaction to direct and consensual light stimulus.
	Eyelid elevation.	Able to retract eyelid fully on command.
	Movement of eye upward and outward, upward, and inward, and medially.	Smooth, symmetrical movements through all six cardinal positions of gaze.
Cranial IV: Trochlear	Movement of eye downward and inward.	
Cranial VI: Abducens	Movement of eye laterally.	

TABLE 17-1: *Continued*

Nerve	Function	Normal Response
Cranial V: Trigeminal	Sensation of face.	Shows brisk blink response to touch of cornea.
	Ophthalmic branch: cornea, ciliary body, conjunctiva, nasal cavity, sinuses; skin of eyebrows, forehead, and nose.	Eyes closed, indicates facial and oral tactile perception. Correctly identifies facial pain stimulus and distinguishes hot and cold applications over three regions.
	Maxillary branch: skin on side of nose, lower eyelid, cheek, upper lip.	
	Mandibular branch: skin of temporal region, external ear, lower face, lower lip, mucosa of anterior 2/3 of tongue, mandibular gums, and the teeth.	
	Movement of muscles of mastication (masseter, temporalis, pterygoideus).	Symmetrical tension in muscles of clenched jaw. Able to move jaw laterally against resistance.
Cranial VII: Facial	Taste to anterior 2/3 of tongue	Perceives sweet, sour, bitter, and salty tastes with each side of anterior tongue.
	Secretion of sublinguinal and submaxillary salivery glands.	
	Movement of facial muscles, scalp, ears, forehead, around eyes, lips.	Able to elevate eyebrows, frown, close eyes tightly, show teeth. With jaw closed, whistle, puff cheeks and smile symmetrically.

111

TABLE 17-1: *Continued*

Nerve	Function	Normal Response
Cranial VIII: Acoustic	Cochlear branch: hearing	With opposite ear masked, hears whispered voice from 2 ft. (60 cm.) and correctly repeats words whispered. With opposite ear masked hears watch tick from same distance at which examiner just able to hear it. Weber: No lateralization Rinne: Air conduction longer than bone conduction Schwabach: Duration of client's bone conduction equal to that of examiner.
	Vestibular branch: balance	Able to tandem walk, stand with feet together without postural deviation. Able to appose finger to nose or finger to finger without past pointing.
Cranial IX: Glosso-pharyngeal	Position of palate and uvula.	Uvula elevates midline.*
	Sensation of mucosa of pharnyx and palatine tonsils. Taste posterior 1/3 of tongue.	Perceives touch stimulus on pharyngeal mucosa.*
	Secretion of parotid salivary gland.	Salivation in response to spicy food.
	Movement of pharynx.	Gag reflex intact.*
Cranial X: Vagus	Movement of palate, pharnyx, and larynx.	Able to phonate without hoarseness or articulation difficulty.

TABLE 17-1: *Continued*

Nerve	Function	Normal Response
		Able to swallow without regurgitating and breathe with ease.
Cranial XI: Accessory	Movement of trapezius and sternocleidomastoid muscles.	Able to raise shoulders against resistance. Able to turn head side to side. Able to strongly oppose resistance to attempt to return chin to midline.
Cranial XII: Hypoglossal	Movement of the tongue.	Tongue protrudes to midline. No tremors, fasciculations, atrophy. Able to oppose resistance. Pronunciation of "R" words intact (e.g. rugged, ragged, third, riding).

*Nerves IX and X both participate in this response.

H. **Sensory assessment?** (NL sensory responses present and symmetrical over all dermatomes and peripheral nerves. Intact light touch, temperature, superficial and deep pain, position, and vibratory senses. Two point discrimination and point localization.) See dermatome map, figure 17-1, and peripheral nerve map, figure 17-2.

I. **Superficial skin, deep tendon, and abnormal reflexes?** Done conventionally with examination of abdomen and extremities. (NL biceps, triceps, brachoradialis, patellar, achilles deep tendon reflexes present; minimal to brisk and symmetrical in intensity. Abdominal, cremasteric, plantar superficial skin reflexes bilaterally intact. No clonus. No pathological reflexes present: Babinski, Chaddock, Hoffman. Evaluation scale for recording reflex intensity: 0 absent, 1+ diminished, 2+ normal, 3+ hyperactive, 4+ hyperactive with clonus.)

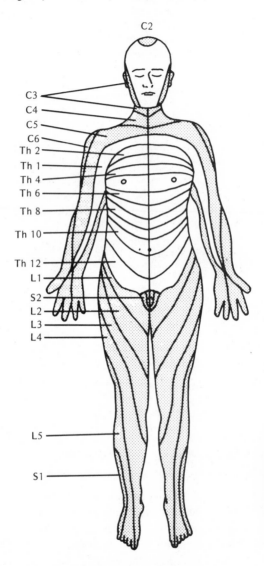

Figure 17-1   Dermatomes

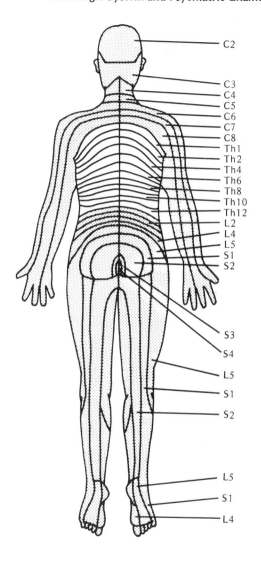

Figure 17-1   *Continued.*

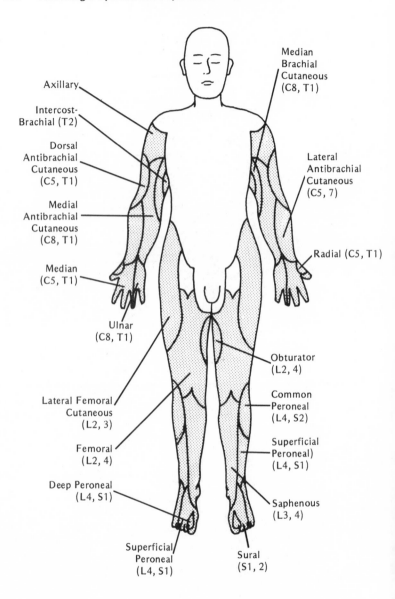

Figure 17-2   Peripheral nerve interruption and sensory loss

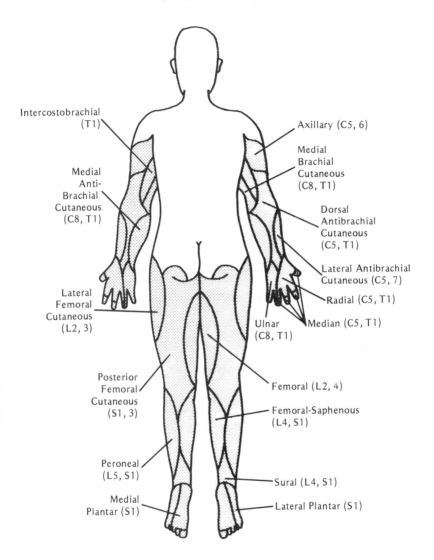

Figure 17-2   *Continued.*

III. LIFE-CYCLE VARIATIONS IN CLINICAL FINDINGS

A. Developmental: Thresholds to touch, pain, and temperature are higher in infancy than in older children and reactions to such stimuli are slower. Deep tendon reflex and plantar responses are variable. Symmetry and consistency of response imply normalcy in infants, as does abatement of infantile reflexes with disappearance at the expected time, and no reemergence or developmental delays. For schedule of reflexes in the infant, see Appendix IX. Assessment of child neurologically involves knowledge of developmental standards. (See emerging patterns of behavior, Appendix VII and VIII, for standard behavior patterns from infancy to age five years.) Development of mental and motor ability after age 5 proceed according to age, educational and cultural enrichment, and physical development endeavors.

B. Degenerative: Loss of brain cells and mass, and increased conduction time of peripheral nerves lead to diminished central and peripheral sensory function, slowing of coordinated movements, and reflex responses. Failing eyesight, reduced hearing and tactile exploration may cause misinterpretation of stimuli. Mental status manifestations of organic brain changes may include rigidity of response, decreased learning capacity, recent memory deficit, and disorientation.

IV. ABNORMAL CONDITIONS

A. Pediatric: Cerebral palsy, dyslexia, encephalitis, epilepsy, hydrocephalus, hyperactivity, hypotonia, meningitis, mental retardation, muscular dystrophy, Von Rechlingshausen's disease.

B. Adult: Amyotrophic lateral sclerosis, brain tumor, cranial neuropathies, herpetic neuropathy, Ménière's syndrome, multiple sclerosis, myesthenia gravis, organic brain syndrome, Parkinson's disease, peripheral neuropathy, postherpetic neuralgia, senile dementia, stroke.

18

Suggested Sequence
of the Physical Examination

A. *Prior to beginning*

1. Assemble equipment.
2. Wash hands.

B. *Approaching the client*

1. Perform measurements: height, weight, blood pressure, respiration, visual acuity, tonometry, audiometry.
2. Request that client (if able) assume a sitting position on bed or table; do the general survey.
3. Take history.

C. *Conducting the remainder of the examination*

1. Stand in front of the client.
   a. Inspect hands and arms.
   b. Palpate hand and arm muscles and joints, check ROM.
   c. Palpate radial pulses.
   d. Move on to head—inspect head and face, check facial movements.
   e. Inspect the eyes, check pupillary reactivity, corneal light reflex, ROM, peripheral vision by confrontation.
   f. Do fundoscopy.
   g. Do informal check of visual acuity (if necessary).
   h. Move to ear—inspect and palpate the right and left pinna.
   i. Do otoscopic examination.

    j.   Conduct tuning fork tests.

    k.   Move to mouth—inspect oral structures and palate, include check of palate movement on phonation, gag reflex, tongue protrusion.

    l.   Check corneal blink reflex and facial sensation.

2.   Stand behind client.

    a.   Inspect neck and spine—check neck ROM, shoulder strength, and movement.

    b.   Palpate neck—check lymph nodes and thyroid.

    c.   Inspect symmetry of chest wall movement and pattern of respiration.

    d.   Palpate vocal fremitus.

    e.   Percuss spine and CVA.

    f.   Percuss posterior lung fields, diaphragm.

    g.   Auscultate posterior lung fields.

3.   Return to front of client who remains in sitting position.

    a.   Inspect anterior neck.

    b.   Palpate carotids and then auscultate them.

    c.   Inspect breasts, axilla, and anterior chest.

    d.   Palpate shoulders, supraclavicular and infraclavicular spaces, ribs, sternum.

    e.   Percuss anterior lung fields.

    f.   Auscultate anterior lung fields.

    g.   Palpate precordium.

    h.   Percuss cardiac borders.

    i.   Auscultate heart sounds.

4.   Stand beside client and have him assume supine position.

    a.   Inspect neck vein pulsation and check neck vein filling.

    b.   Palpate breasts.

    c.   Repeat cardiac auscultation in left lateral position.

    d.   Have patient return to supine position—inspect abdomen and flanks.

    e.   Auscultate bowel sounds, abdominal bruits.

    f.   Percuss the liver and spleen.

    g.   Check abdominal skin reflexes.

h. Do light and deep palpation of abdominal quadrants, bimanual palpation of liver, spleen, and kidneys.

i. Inspect inguinal region.

j. Palpate and auscultate femoral arteries.

k. Inspect legs, check ROM, and muscle strength.

l. Palpate joints of lower extremity, palpate leg and foot pulses.

m. Test touch, pain, temperature, and vibratory senses over abdomen and legs.

n. Inspect and palpate genitalia.

    1. Conduct speculum and bimanual pelvic examination on female—checking rectum.

    2. Conduct cremasteric reflex in male.

5. Stand in front of client and have him assume sitting position.

  a. Check deep tendon reflexes, Babinski, position sense of feet.

  b. Check past-pointing, alternating movements.

6. Have client assume standing position.

  a. Check Romberg, tandem walking, heel and toe walking, deep knee bending (if possible).

  b. Do hernia check on male client, then have him bend at waist for rectal examination.

Appendices

APPENDIX I: HEIGHT AND WEIGHT TABLES FOR ADULTS

Desirable weights for persons age 25 and over in pounds according to frame, wearing indoor clothing

FOR MEN 25 YEARS OF AGE OR OLDER

HEIGHT[a] Feet	Inches	SMALL FRAME	MEDIUM FRAME	LARGE FRAME
5	2	112-120	118-129	126-141
5	3	115-123	121-133	129-144
5	4	118-126	124-136	132-148
5	5	121-129	127-139	135-152
5	6	124-133	130-143	138-156
5	7	128-137	134-147	142-161
5	8	132-141	138-152	147-166
5	9	136-145	142-156	151-170
5	10	140-150	146-160	155-174
5	11	144-154	150-165	159-179
6	0	148-158	154-170	164-184
6	1	152-162	158-175	168-189
6	2	156-167	162-180	173-194
6	3	160-171	167-185	178-199
6	4	164-175	172-190	182-204

a. with shoes on, 1-inch heels

FOR WOMEN 25 YEARS OF AGE OR OLDER

HEIGHT[b] Feet	Inches	SMALL FRAME	MEDIUM FRAME	LARGE FRAME
4	10	92- 98	96-107	104-119
4	11	94-101	98-110	106-122
5	0	96-104	101-113	109-125
5	1	99-107	104-116	112-128
5	2	102-110	107-119	115-131
5	3	105-113	110-122	118-134
5	4	108-116	113-126	121-138
5	5	111-119	116-130	125-142
5	6	114-123	120-135	129-146
5	7	118-127	124-139	133-150
5	8	122-131	128-143	137-154
5	9	126-135	132-147	141-158
5	10	130-140	136-151	145-163
5	11	134-144	140-155	149-168
6	0	138-148	144-159	153-173

b. with shoes on, 2-inch heels

SOURCE: C. H. Robinson with M. R. Lawlor, *Normal and Therapeutic Nutrition*, 14th ed, Macmillan, New York, 1972, p. 703

APPENDIX II: PHYSICAL GROWTH

Age		PERCENTILES, BOYS								PERCENTILES, GIRLS						
		5th	10th	25th	50th	75th	90th	95th		5th	10th	25th	50th	75th	90th	95th
AT BIRTH	Length-cm.	46.4	47.5	49.0	50.5	51.8	53.5	54.4		45.4	46.5	48.2	49.9	51.0	52.0	52.9
	Length-in.	18¼	18¾	19¼	20	20½	21	21½		17¾	18¼	19	19¾	20	20½	20¾
	Weight-kg.	2.54	2.78	3.00	3.27	3.64	3.82	4.15		2.36	2.58	2.93	3.23	3.52	3.64	3.81
	Weight-lb.	5½	6¼	6½	7¼	8	8½	9¼		5¼	5¾	6½	7	7¾	8	8½
	Head C-cm.	32.6	33.0	33.9	34.8	35.6	36.6	37.2		32.1	32.9	33.5	34.3	34.8	35.5	35.9
	Head C-in.	12¾	13	13¾	13¾	14	14½	14¾		12¾	13	13¾	13½	13¾	14	14¼
3 MONTHS	Length-cm.	56.7	57.7	59.4	61.1	63.0	64.5	65.4		55.4	56.2	57.8	59.5	61.2	62.7	63.4
	Length-in.	22¼	22¾	23½	24	24¾	25¼	25¾		21¾	22¼	22¾	23½	24	24¾	25
	Weight-kg.	4.43	4.78	5.32	5.98	6.56	7.14	7.37		4.18	4.47	4.88	5.40	5.90	6.39	6.74
	Weight-lb.	9¾	10½	11¾	13¼	14½	15¾	16¼		9¼	9¾	10¾	12	13	14	14¾
	Head C-cm.	38.4	38.9	39.7	40.6	41.7	42.5	43.1		37.3	37.8	38.7	39.5	40.4	41.2	41.7
	Head C-in.	15	15¼	15¾	16	16½	16¾	17		14¾	15	15¼	15½	16	16¼	16½
6 MONTHS	Length-cm.	63.4	64.4	66.1	67.8	69.7	71.3	72.3		61.8	62.6	64.2	65.9	67.8	69.4	70.2
	Length-in.	25	25¼	26	26¾	27½	28	28½		24¼	24¾	25¼	26	26¾	27¼	27¾
	Weight-kg.	6.20	6.61	7.20	7.85	8.49	9.10	9.46		5.79	6.12	6.60	7.21	7.83	8.38	8.73
	Weight-lb.	13¾	14½	15¾	17¼	18¾	20	20¾		12¾	13½	14½	16	17¼	18½	19¼
	Head C-cm.	41.5	42.0	42.8	43.8	44.7	45.6	46.2		40.3	40.9	41.6	42.4	43.3	44.1	44.6
	Head C-in.	16¼	16½	16¾	17¼	17½	18	18¼		15¾	16	16½	16¾	17	17¼	17½

12 MONTHS													
Length-cm.	81.2	79.8	77.7	76.1	74.3	72.8	71.7	69.8	70.8	72.4	74.3	76.3	78.0	79.1
Length-in.	32	31½	30½	30	29¼	28¾	28¼	27½	27¾	28½	29¼	30	30¾	31¼
Weight-kg.	11.99	11.54	10.91	10.15	9.49	8.84	8.43	7.84	8.19	8.81	9.53	10.23	10.87	11.24
Weight-lb.	26½	25½	24	22½	21	19½	18½	17¼	18	19½	21	22½	24	24¾
Head C-cm.	49.3	48.8	47.9	47.0	46.1	45.3	44.8	43.5	44.1	44.8	45.6	46.4	47.2	47.6
Head C-in.	19½	19¼	18¾	18½	18¼	17¾	17¾	17¼	17¼	17¾	18	18¼	18½	18¾
18 MONTHS													
Length-cm.	88.1	86.6	84.3	82.4	80.5	78.7	77.5	76.0	77.2	78.8	80.9	83.0	85.0	86.1
Length-in.	34¾	34	33¼	32½	31¾	31	30½	30	30½	31	31¾	32½	33½	34
Weight-kg.	13.44	13.05	12.31	11.47	10.67	9.92	9.59	8.92	9.30	10.04	10.82	11.55	12.30	12.76
Weight-lb.	29½	28¾	27¼	25¼	23½	21¾	21¼	19¾	20½	22¼	23¾	25½	27	28¼
Head C-cm.	50.6	50.1	49.3	48.4	47.4	46.7	46.3	45.0	45.6	46.3	47.1	47.9	48.6	49.1
Head C-in.	20	19¾	19½	19	18¾	18½	18¼	17¾	18	18¼	18½	18¾	19¼	19¼
24 MONTHS													
Length-cm.	93.8	92.2	89.9	87.6	85.6	83.5	82.3	81.3	82.5	84.2	86.5	88.7	90.8	92.0
Length-in.	37	36¼	35½	34½	33¾	32¾	32½	32	32½	33¼	34	35	35½	36¼
Weight-kg.	14.70	14.29	13.44	12.59	11.65	10.85	10.54	9.87	10.26	11.10	11.90	12.74	13.57	14.08
Weight-lb.	32½	31½	29½	27¾	25¾	24	23¼	21¾	22½	24½	26¼	28	30	31
Head C-cm.	51.4	51.0	50.2	49.2	48.3	47.7	47.3	46.1	46.5	47.3	48.1	48.8	49.6	50.1
Head C-in.	20¼	20	19¾	19¼	19	18¾	18½	18¼	18¼	18½	19	19¼	19½	19¾
36 MONTHS													
Length-cm.	103.1	101.4	98.9	96.5	94.2	92.4	91.2	90.0	91.0	93.1	95.6	98.1	100.1	101.5
Length-in.	40½	40	39	38	37	36½	36	35½	35¾	36¾	37¾	38½	39½	40
Weight-kg.	17.28	16.66	15.59	14.69	13.58	12.69	12.26	11.60	12.07	12.99	13.93	15.03	15.97	16.54
Weight-lb.	38	36¾	34¼	32½	30	28	27	25½	26½	28¾	30¾	33¼	35¼	36½
Head C-cm.	52.8	52.3	51.5	50.5	49.7	49	48.6	47.6	47.9	48.5	49.3	50.0	50.8	51.4
Head C-in.	20¾	20½	20¼	19¾	19½	19¼	19¼	18¾	18¾	19	19½	19¾	20	20¼

National Center for Health Statistics, Health Resources Administration, D.H.E.W., Hyattsville, Md. Data from Fels Research Institute, Yellow Springs, Ohio; smoothed by least squares-cubic-spline technique. Conversion of metric data to inches and pounds by Ross Laboratories.

APPENDIX II: PHYSICAL GROWTH

	PERCENTILES, BOYS								PERCENTILES, GIRLS						
Age	*5th*	*10th*	*25th*	*50th*	*75th*	*90th*	*95th*		*5th*	*10th*	*25th*	*50th*	*75th*	*90th*	*95th*
4	**95.8**	**97.3**	**100.0**	**102.9**	**105.7**	**108.2**	**109.9**	**Stature-cm.**	**95.0**	**96.4**	**98.8**	**101.6**	**104.3**	**106.6**	**108.3**
YEARS	37¾	38¼	39¼	40½	41½	42½	43¼	Stature-in.	37½	38	39	40	41	42	42¾
	13.64	**14.24**	**15.39**	**16.69**	**17.99**	**19.32**	**20.27**	**Weight-kg.**	**13.11**	**13.84**	**14.80**	**15.96**	**17.56**	**18.93**	**19.91**
	30	31½	34	36¾	39¾	42½	44¾	Weight-lbs.	29	30½	32¾	35¼	38¾	41¾	44
5	**102.0**	**103.7**	**106.5**	**109.9**	**112.8**	**115.4**	**117.0**	**Stature-cm.**	**101.1**	**102.7**	**105.4**	**108.4**	**111.4**	**113.8**	**115.6**
YEARS	40¼	40¾	42	43¼	44½	45½	46	Stature-in.	39¾	40½	41½	42¾	43¾	44¾	45½
	15.27	**15.96**	**17.22**	**18.67**	**20.14**	**21.70**	**23.09**	**Weight-kg.**	**14.55**	**15.26**	**16.29**	**17.66**	**19.39**	**21.23**	**22.62**
	33¾	35¼	38	41¼	44½	47¾	51	Weight-lbs.	32	33¾	36	39	42¾	46¾	49¾
6	**107.7**	**109.6**	**112.5**	**116.1**	**119.2**	**121.9**	**123.5**	**Stature-cm.**	**106.6**	**108.4**	**111.3**	**114.6**	**118.1**	**120.8**	**122.7**
YEARS	42½	43¼	44¼	45¾	47	48	48½	Stature-in.	42	42¾	43¾	45	46½	47½	48¼
	16.93	**17.72**	**19.07**	**20.69**	**22.40**	**24.31**	**26.34**	**Weight-kg.**	**16.05**	**16.72**	**17.86**	**19.52**	**21.44**	**23.89**	**25.75**
	37¼	39	42	45½	49½	53½	58	Weight-lbs.	35½	36¾	39¼	43	47¼	52¾	56¾
8	**118.1**	**120.2**	**123.2**	**127.0**	**130.5**	**133.6**	**135.7**	**Stature-cm.**	**116.9**	**118.7**	**122.2**	**126.4**	**130.6**	**134.2**	**136.2**
YEARS	46½	47¼	48½	50	51½	52½	53½	Stature-in.	46	46¾	48	49¾	51½	52¾	53½
	20.40	**21.39**	**23.09**	**25.30**	**27.91**	**31.06**	**34.51**	**Weight-kg.**	**19.62**	**20.45**	**22.26**	**24.84**	**27.88**	**32.04**	**34.71**
	45	47¼	51	55¾	61½	68½	76	Weight-lbs.	43¼	45	49	54¾	61½	70¾	76½

10	**127.7**	**130.1**	**133.4**	**137.5**	**141.6**	**145.5**	**148.1**	**Stature-cm.**	**127.5**	**129.5**	**133.6**	**138.3**	**142.9**	**147.2**	**149.5**
YEARS	50¼	51¼	52½	54¼	55¾	57¼	58¼	Stature-in.	50¼	51	52½	54½	56¼	58	58¾
	24.33	**25.52**	**28.07**	**31.44**	**35.61**	**40.80**	**45.27**	**Weight-kg.**	**24.36**	**25.76**	**28.71**	**32.55**	**37.53**	**43.70**	**47.17**
	53¾	56¼	62	69¼	78½	90	99¾	Weight-lbs.	53¾	56¾	63¼	71¾	82¾	96¼	104
12	**137.6**	**140.3**	**144.4**	**149.7**	**154.6**	**159.4**	**162.3**	**Stature-cm.**	**139.8**	**142.3**	**147.0**	**151.5**	**155.8**	**160.0**	**162.7**
YEARS	54¼	55¼	56¾	59	60¾	62¾	64	Stature-in.	55	56	57¾	59¾	61¼	63	64
	29.85	**31.46**	**35.09**	**39.78**	**45.77**	**52.73**	**58.09**	**Weight-kg.**	**30.52**	**32.53**	**36.52**	**41.53**	**48.07**	**55.99**	**60.81**
	65¾	69¼	77¼	87¾	101	116¼	128	Weight-lbs.	67¼	71¾	80½	91½	106	123½	134
14	**148.8**	**151.8**	**156.9**	**163.1**	**168.5**	**173.8**	**176.7**	**Stature-cm.**	**148.7**	**151.5**	**155.9**	**160.4**	**164.6**	**168.7**	**171.3**
YEARS	58½	59¾	61¾	64¼	66¼	68½	69½	Stature-cm.	58½	59¾	61½	63¼	64¾	66½	67½
	38.22	**40.64**	**45.21**	**50.77**	**58.31**	**65.57**	**72.13**	**Weight-kg.**	**37.76**	**40.11**	**44.54**	**50.28**	**57.09**	**66.04**	**73.08**
	84¼	89½	99¾	112	128½	144½	159	Weight-lbs.	83¼	88½	98¼	110¾	125¾	145½	161
16	**161.1**	**163.9**	**168.7**	**173.5**	**178.1**	**182.4**	**185.4**	**Stature-cm.**	**151.6**	**154.1**	**157.8**	**162.4**	**166.9**	**171.1**	**173.3**
YEARS	63½	64½	66½	68¼	70	71¾	73	Stature-in.	59¾	60¾	62¼	64	65¾	67¼	68¼
	47.74	**51.16**	**56.16**	**62.10**	**70.26**	**77.97**	**85.62**	**Weight-kg.**	**43.41**	**45.78**	**50.09**	**55.89**	**62.29**	**71.68**	**80.99**
	105¼	112¾	123¾	137	155	172	188¾	Weight-lbs.	95¾	101	110½	123¼	137¼	158	178½
18	**165.7**	**168.7**	**172.3**	**176.8**	**181.2**	**185.3**	**187.6**	**Stature-cm.**	**153.6**	**156.0**	**159.6**	**163.7**	**167.6**	**171.0**	**173.6**
YEARS	65¼	66½	67¾	69½	71¼	73	73¾	Stature-in.	60½	61½	62¾	64½	66	67¼	68¼
	53.97	**57.89**	**62.61**	**68.88**	**76.04**	**88.41**	**95.76**	**Weight-kg.**	**45.26**	**47.47**	**51.39**	**56.62**	**62.78**	**72.25**	**82.47**
	119	127¼	138	151¾	167¾	195	211	Weight-lbs.	99¾	104¾	113¼	124¾	138½	159¼	181¾

National Center for Health Statistics, Health Resources Administration, D.H.E.W., Hyattsville, Maryland 20782. Data from N.C.H.S. National Health Surveys, smoothed by least-square-cubic-spline technique. Conversion of metric data to inches and pounds by Ross Laboratories.

APPENDIX III
NORMAL RANGES OF ARTERIAL BLOOD PRESSURE IN ADULTS*

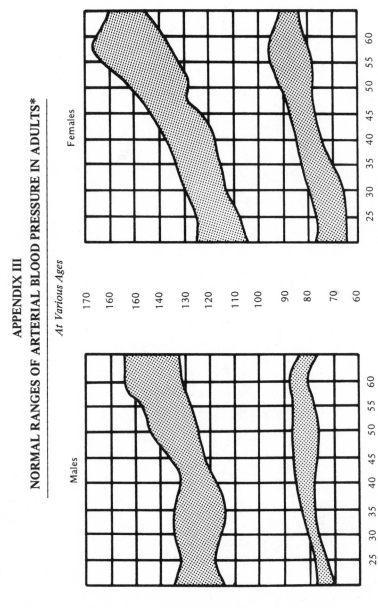

At Various Ages

Males   Females

* Altma, Philip L, Dorothy S. Ditmer, *Respiration and Circulation*, Bethesda, Md.: Federation of American Societies

APPENDIX IV
NORMAL RANGES OF ARTERIAL BLOOD PRESSURE IN CHILDREN

Ages	Mean Systolic ± 2 S.D.	Mean Diastolic ± 2 S.D.
Newborn	80 ± 16	46 ± 16
6–12 months	89 ± 29	60 ± 10
1 year	96 ± 30	66 ± 25
2 years	99 ± 25	64 ± 25
3 years	100 ± 25	67 ± 23
4 years	99 ± 20	65 ± 20
5–6 years	94 ± 14	55 ± 9
6–7 years	100 ± 15	56 ± 8
8–9 years	105 ± 16	57 ± 9
9–10 years	107 ± 16	57 ± 9
10–11 years	111 ± 17	58 ± 10
11–12 years	113 ± 18	59 ± 10
12 –13 years	115 ± 19	59 ± 10
13–14 years	118 ± 19	60 ± 10

R. J. Haggerty, M. W. Maroney, and A. S. Nadas, "Essential hypertension in infancy and childhood," *A.M.A.J. Dis. Child,* 92:536, 1956. Copyright 1956, American Medical Association.

APPENDIX V
NORMAL PULSE RATES FOR VARIOUS AGES

AGE	PULSE RATES
Newborn	110–150
11 months	100–140
2 years	90–110
4 years	80–120
6 years	80–100
8 years	76–90
10 years	70–110
Adult	60–100

APPENDIX VI
NORMAL RESPIRATORY RATES FOR VARIOUS AGES

AGE	RESPIRATORY RATE
Neonate	30–50
2 years	20–30
10 years	14–22
Adolescent	12–20
Adult	12–20

APPENDIX VII
EMERGING PATTERNS OF BEHAVIOR DURING THE FIRST YEAR OF LIFE

NEONATAL PERIOD (FIRST 4 WEEKS)

Prone: Lies in flexed attitude; turns head from side to side; head sags on ventral suspension

Supine: Generally flexed and a little stiff

Visual: May fixate face of light in line of vision "doll's eye" movement of eyes on turning of the body

Reflex: Moro response active; stepping and placing reflexes; grasp reflex active

AT 4 WEEKS

Prone: Legs more extended; holds chin up; turns head; head lifted momentarily to plane of body on ventral suspension

Supine: Tonic neck posture predominates; supple and relaxed; head lags on pull to sitting position

Visual: Watches person; follows moving object a few degrees

AT 8 WEEKS

Prone: Raises head slightly farther; head sustained in plane of body on ventral suspension

Supine: Tonic neck posture predominates; head lags on pull to sitting position

Visual: Follows moving object 180 degrees

Social: Smiles on social contact; listens to voice and coos

Prone: Lifts head and chest, arms extended; head above plane of body on ventral suspension

Supine: Tonic neck posture predominates; reaches toward and misses objects; waves at toy

Sitting: Head lag partially compensated on pull to sitting position; early head control with bobbing motion; back rounded

Reflex: Typical Moro response has not persisted; makes defense movements or selective withdrawal reactions

Social: Sustained social contact; listens to music; says "aah, ngah"

Prone: Lifts head and chest, head in approximately vertical axis; legs extended

Supine: Symmetrical posture predominates, hands in midline; reaches and grasps objects and brings them to mouth

Sitting: No head lag on pull to sitting position; head steady, held forward; enjoys sitting with full truncal support

Standing: When held erect, pushes with feet

Adaptive: Sees pellet, but makes no move to it

Social: Laughs out loud; may show displeasure if social contact is broken; excited at sight of food

Prone: Rolls over; may pivot

Supine: Lifts head; rolls over; squirming movements

Sitting: Sits briefly, with support of pelvis; leans forward on hands; back rounded

Standing: May support most of weight; bounces actively

Adaptive: Reaches out for and grasps large object; transfers objects from hand to hand; grasp uses radial palm; rakes at pellet

Language: Polysyllabic vowel sounds formed

Social: Prefers mother; babbles; enjoys mirror; responds to changes in emotional content of social contact

AT 40 WEEKS

Sitting:	Sits up alone and indefinitely without support, back straight
Standing:	Pulls to standing position
Motor:	Creeps or crawls
Adaptive:	Grasps objects with thumb and forefinger; pokes at things with forefinger; picks up pellet with assisted pincer movement; uncovers hidden toy; attempts to retrieve dropped object; releases object grasped by other person
Language:	Repetitive consonant sounds (mama, dada)
Social:	Responds to sound of name; plays peek-a-boo or pat-a-cake; waves bye-bye

AT 52 WEEKS (1 YEAR)

Motor:	Walks with one hand held; "cruises" or walks holding on to furniture
Adaptive:	Picks up pellet with unassisted pincer movement of forefinger and thumb; releases object to other person on request or gesture
Language:	2 "words" besides mama, dada
Social:	Plays simple ball game; makes postural adjustment to dressing

V. Vaughan, and R. J. McKay, editors, *Nelson Textbook of Pediatrics*, 10th ed., W. B. Saunders Co., Philadelphia, 1975, p. 49.

APPENDIX VIII
EMERGING PATTERNS OF BEHAVIOR FROM 1 to 5 YEARS OF AGE

15 MONTHS

Motor:	Walks alone; crawls up stairs
Adaptive:	Makes tower of 2 cubes; makes a line with crayon; inserts pellet in bottle
Language:	Jargon; follows simple commands; may name a familiar object (ball)
Social:	Indicates some desires or needs by pointing

18 MONTHS

Motor:	Runs stiffly; sits on small chair; walks up stairs with one hand held; explores drawers and waste baskets
Adaptive:	Piles 3 cubes; imitates scribbling; imitates vertical stroke; dumps pellet from bottle
Language:	10 words (average); names pictures
Social:	Feeds self; seeks help when in trouble; may complain when wet or soiled

24 MONTHS

Motor:	Runs well; walks up and down stairs, one step at a time; opens doors; climbs on furniture
Adaptive:	Tower of 6 cubes; circular scribbling; imitates horizontal stroke; folds paper once imitatively
Language:	Puts 3 words together (pronoun, verb, object)
Social:	Handles spoon well; often tells immediate experiences; helps to undress; listens to stories with pictures

30 MONTHS

Motor:	Jumps
Adaptive:	Tower of 8 cubes; makes vertical and horizontal strokes, but generally will not join them to make a cross; imitates circular stroke, forming closed figure
Language:	Refers to self by pronoun "I"; knows full name
Social:	Helps put things away

36 MONTHS

Motor:	Goes up stairs alternating feet; rides tricycle; stands momentarily on one foot
Adaptive:	Tower of 9 cubes; imitates construction of "bridge" of 3 cubes; copies a circle; imitates a cross
Language:	Knows age and sex; counts 3 objects correctly; repeats 3 numbers or a sentence of 6 syllables
Social:	Plays simple games (in "parallel" with other children); helps in dressing (unbuttons clothing and puts on shoes); washes hands

48 MONTHS

Motor:	Hops on one foot; throws ball overhand; uses scissors to cut out pictures; climbs well
Adaptive:	Copies bridge from model; imitates construction of "gate" of 5 cubes; copies cross and square; draws a man with 2 to 4 parts besides head; names longer of 2 lines
Language:	Counts 4 pennies accurately; tells a story
Social:	Plays with several children with beginning of social interaction and role-playing; goes to toilet alone

60 MONTHS

Motor:	Skips
Adaptive:	Draws triangle from copy; names heavier of 2 weights
Language:	Names 4 colors; repeats sentence of 10 syllables; counts 10 pennies correctly
Social:	Dresses and undresses; asks questions about meaning of words; domestic role-playing

After 5 years the Stanford-Binet, Wechsler-Bellevue, and other scales offer the most precise estimates of developmental level. In order to have their greatest value, they should be administered only by an experienced and qualified person.

V. Vaughan and R. J. McKay, editors. *Nelson Textbook of Pediatrics.* 10th ed. Philadelphia: W. B. Saunders Co., 1975, p. 50.

APPENDIX IX
SCHEDULE OF REFLEXES IN THE INFANT

Reflex	Normal Response	Appearance	Disappearance
1. Plantar	Both extension and flexion of toes in response to firm lateral plantar stroke, with extension predominating. May be associated with leg withdrawal.	Variable	End of 2nd year
2. Palmar Grasp	Gripping of examiner's finger in response to light pressure on infant's palm, with tightening of grip on any attempt to remove finger.	Birth	2nd to 4th month
3. Rooting	In response to touch of cheek, turns head toward stimulus and opens mouth.	Birth	3-4 months awake, 7 months asleep
4. Sucking	Sucking movements in response to stimulation of the lips.	Birth	3-4 months awake, 7 months asleep
5. Moro	Abduction and extension of all four extremities in response to sudden stimulus (such as loud noise) followed by adduction and flexion.	Birth	Before 5th month

Reflex	Normal Response	Appear-ance	Disappear-ance
6. Stepping	Movements of progression in response to being held upright and slightly forward with soles of feet touching a flat surface.	Birth	6 weeks
7. Placing	Flexion followed by extension of the leg in response to drawing the dorsum of the foot along the under edge of a table top while the infant is held in the erect position.	Birth	6 weeks
8. Tonic Neck	In response to rapidly turning head to side, arm and leg on side toward which head is turned are extended.	Birth to 2 months	6 months
9. Neck Righting	Rotation of the trunk in direction in which the head of the supine infant is turned.	4–6 months	24 months
10. Landau	In prone position, with examiner's hand supporting infant at the abdomen, infant extends head, trunk and hips. On flexing the head, flexion of trunk and hips follows.	3 months	24 months

Reflex	*Normal Response*	*Appearance*	*Disappearance*
11. Acoustic Blink	A blink or contraction of the eyelids in response to loud, sudden noise.	Birth— may be difficult to elicit on days 1-3, possibly due to lack of air in middle ear.	Variable
12. Optic Blink	Firm contraction of eyelids, and sometimes quick dorsiflexion of head in response to sudden light shined in eyes.	Birth	Blink persists through life. Head dorsiflexion disappears by 5th month.
13. Abdominal	Prompt retraction of abdominal skin on same side in response to touch stimulus in area of umbilicus. May take form of mass reaction.	Age 6 months	Persists through life
14. Cremasteric	Elevation of scrotum and testes on same side in response to touching thigh.	Age 6 months	Persists through life

Reflex	Normal Response	Appear-ance	Disappear-ance
15. Deep Tendon	Prompt contraction of corresponding muscle in response to tap of tendon.	Most present at birth. Triceps reflex may not appear until 6 months of age.	Persists through life

Abbreviations

A	aortic	**Gen**	general
AAL	anterior axillary line	**GEO**	geographic
ADL	activities of daily living	**GI**	gastrointestinal
AGE	angle of greatest extension	**gm**	gram
		GU	genitourinary
AGF	angle of greatest flexion	**HEENT**	head, eyes, ears, nose, and throat
A-P diam	anterior-posterior diameter	**H&P**	history and physical
ARDS	adult respiratory distress syndrome	**HPI**	history of present illness
ausc	auscultation	**Ht**	height
A-V	arteriovenous	**Hx**	history
A&W	alive and well	**ICS**	intercostal space
BP	blood pressure	**ID**	identifying information
CC	chief complaint	**insp**	inspection
cm	centimeter	**kg**	kilogram
CN	cranial nerve		
CV	cardiovascular	**L**	left
CVA	costovertebral angle	**LAAL**	left anterior axillary line
Dx	diagnosis	**LBCD**	left border cardiac dullness
DPT	diphtheria, pertussis, tetanus	**LICS**	left intercostal space
		LLQ	left lower quadrant
EENT	eyes, ears, nose, and throat	**LLSB**	lower left sternal border
EOM	extra ocular movements	**LMP**	last menstrual period
F	father	**LOC**	level of consciousness
FH	family history		

LRSB	lower right sternal border	**Psych**	psychiatric
LSB	left sternal border	**Pt**	patient
LUQ	left upper quadrant	**R**	right
M	mother, mitral	**RAAL**	right anterior axillary line
marit	marital	**RICS**	right intercostal space
MAL	midaxillary line	**RLQ**	right lower quadrant
MCL	midclavicular line	**ROM**	range of motion
mg	milligram	**ROS**	review of systems
MIL	midinguinal line	**RSB**	right sternal border
mm	millimeter	**RUQ**	right upper quadrant
MMR	measles, mumps, rubella	**Rx**	treatment
MS	musculoskeletal	S_1	first heart sound
MSL	midsternal line, mid-scapular line	S_2	second heart sound
		S_3	third heart sound
nl, NL	normal	S_4	fourth heart sound
NP	neuropsychiatric	**SH**	social history
N&V	nausea and vomiting	**SOB**	shortness of breath
OB	obstetrical	**T**	tricuspid
OD	right eye	**TB**	tuberculosis
OS	left eye	**TM**	tympanic membrane
OU	both eyes	**TOPV**	trivalent oral polio vaccine
P	pulmonic	**TPR**	temperature, pulse, respiration
PAL	posterior axillary line		
palp	palpation	**ULSB**	upper left sternal border
Pap	pap smear		
perc	percussion	**URI**	upper respiratory infection
PERRLA	pupils equal, round, reactive to light and accommodation	**URSB**	upper right sternal border
PMH	past medical history	**WNL**	within normal limits
PMI	point of maximal impulse or intensity	**Wt**	weight
P/SH	personal and social history		

References

Alexander, Mary, and Marie Brown, *Pediatric History Taking and Physical Diagnosis for Nurses,* 2nd ed., McGraw-Hill, New York, 1979

Andreoli, Kathleen, Virginia Hunn Fowkes, Douglas Zipes, and Andrew Wallace, *Comprehensive Cardiac Care*, 3rd ed., C. V. Mosby, St. Louis, 1975.

Bates, Barbara, *Guide to Physical Examination*, 2nd ed., J. B. Lippincott, Philadelphia, 1979.

Caird, F. I., and T. G. Judge, *Assessment of the Elderly Patient*, Pitman Publishing, New York, 1974.

Capell, Peter, and David Case, *Ambulatory Care Manual for Nurse Practitioners*, J. B. Lippincott, Philadelphia, 1976.

Cherniack, Reuben, Louis Cherniack, and Arnold Naimark, *Respiration in Health and Disease*, 2nd ed., W. B. Saunders, Philadelphia, 1972.

Chinn, Austin, *Working with Older People: Clinical Aspects of Aging*, U.S. Department of Health, Education, and Welfare, Rockville, Md., 1971.

Degowin, Elmer, and Richard Degowin, *Bedside Diagnostic Examination*, Macmillan, New York, 1976.

Delp, Mahlon, and R. T. Manning, *Majors Physical Diagnosis*, 8th ed., W. B. Saunders, Philadelphia, 1975.

Gilles, Dee Ann, and Irene Alyn, *Patient Assessment and Management by the Nurse Practitioner*, W. B. Saunders, Philadelphia, 1976.

Johnson, Thomas, William Moore, and James Jeffries, editors, *Children Are Different: Developmental Physiology,* Ross Laboratories, Columbus, Ohio, 1978.

Judge, Richard, and George Zuidema, editors, *Methods of Clinical Examination: A Physiologic Approach*, 3rd ed., Little, Brown, Boston, 1974.

Malasanos, Lois, Violet Barkouskas, Muriel Moss, Kathryn Stollenberg-Allen, *Health Assessment*, C. V. Mosby, St. Louis, 1977.

Pansky, Ben, and Earl Lawrence House, *Review of Gross Anatomy*, 3rd ed., Macmillan, New York, 1975.

Patton, Harry O., John W. Sundsten, Wayne E. Crill, Phillip D. Swanson, *Introduction to Basic Neurology*, W. B. Saunders, Philadelphia, 1976.

Prior, John, and Jack Silberstein, *Physical Diagnosis*, 5th ed., W. B. Saunders, Philadelphia, 1977.

Rossman, Isador, editor, *Clinical Geriatrics*, J. B. Lippincott, Philadelphia, 1971.

Sherman, Jacques, and Sylvia Fields, *Guide to Patient Evaluation*, 2nd ed., Medical Examination Publishing, Flushing, New York, 1976.

Steinberg, Franz, editor, *Cowdry's The Care of the Geriatric Patient*, C. V. Mosby, St. Louis, 1976.

Vaugh, Victor, and James McKay, editors, *Nelson Textbook of Pediatrics*, 10th ed., W. B. Saunders, Philadelphia, 1975.

PHYSICAL EXAMINATION AT A GLANCE

MEASUREMENTS: Ht., wt., BP, TPR, tonometry, visual acuity, audiometry.

GENERAL SURVEY: Mental status; appearance; apparent sex, race, age; nutrition; body development, proportions; station/posture; movement/gait; dominance; energy; speech; odors.

INTEGUMENT: Skin color, texture, temperature, turgor, hygiene, veins, lesions, masses, edema; hair; nails.

HEAD, SKULL, SCALP, FACE: Size, contour, hygiene, proportions, pigmentation, expression, movement, sensation, edema, masses, lesions, lymph nodes, tenderness.

EYE: Brows and lashes; lid conformation position, blinking, inflammation, lesions, tearing, eyeball/orbit; conjunctiva color, moisture, lesions; sclera color; cornea color, contour, depth, sensitivity; iris color, shape; pupil shape, size, reactivity; eye alignment; extraocular movement; red reflex; disc shape, size, margins, color, cup-to-disc ratio; retinal vessels; ocular tension, compressibility; visual acuity, color vision, near vision, visual fields.

EAR: Pinna shape, position, tenderness; mastoid tenderness; auditory canal malformation, cerumen, foreign body, lesion; TM landmarks; hearing voice, watch tick, tuning fork tests.

NOSE, MOUTH, THROAT: Turbinates; septal deviation; mucosal moisture; lips movement, condition; teeth; gum condition; tongue texture, size, movement; sublingual veins; oral mucosal texture; salivary duct patency; palate contour, movement; uvula; tonsils size, contour, membrane; posterior pharyngeal wall edema, discharge, movement; sinus tenderness; smell; taste; voice quality; color and lesions of all tissues.

NECK: Symmetry, curvature, ROM, head movement, pulsation, lymph nodes, venous distension, thyroid enlargement, masses; tracheal position; muscle strength.

BREASTS, AXILLAE: Breasts—size, symmetry, color, contour, hair pattern, venous pattern, edema, lesions, scars, rashes, masses, retractions pre-menstrual changes, tenderness; areola—color; nipple—lesions, discharge retractions; axilla—hair distribution, rashes, ulcers, masses, tenderness.

CHEST: Coutour, dimensions, rib angle, movement; skin color, moisture scars; respiratory rate, rhythm, depth, quality, type, ratio to heart rate